D1084725

Being Fit:
A Personal Guide

**Bud Getchell
with
Wayne Anderson**

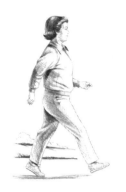

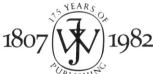

175 YEARS OF
1807 WJ 1982
PUBLISHING

John Wiley & Sons, Inc.
New York • Chichester • Brisbane • Toronto • Singapore

Library of Congress Cataloging in Publication Data

Getchell, Bud,   1934 -
    Being fit.

    Includes index.
    1. Exercise   2. Physical fitness.
I. Anderson, Wayne, 1941 -   . II. Title.
RA781.G46   613.7'1   81-23079
ISBN 0-471-86353-X   AACR2

Printed in the United States of America

83   82   10   9   8   7   6   5   4   3   2   1

Contents

Foreword

Anyone who makes a study, as I have, of the physical fitness literature knows how tediously repetitious so much of it is. And no wonder. Many writers on the subject have had little or no practical experience. They have, it is true, done their homework in the library, but too often they have not done much else.

Bud Getchell, the principal author of this book, is different. A former college athlete (and All-American second baseman), he is the founder and currently a staff member of Ball State University's Human Performance Laboratory, where for several years he has directed a much-imitated physical fitness program for adults. Most impressive of all, Getchell is an unswerving realist who acknowledges that exercise, even for the most committed enthusiast, is not invariably unalloyed joy and that finding time for it can be a vexation. "Our modern life-style fosters unfitness," he writes. "We have become accustomed to riding, sitting, and watching."

These are the enemies. This, therefore, is a book for busy people living in a society that does not, despite recent advances, offer much applause or even respectful tolerance for those of us who want to take good care of ourselves. It is a wise and practical work and one that, if steadfastly followed, cannot help but bring a great many benefits.

Bud Getchell, I am glad to report, is no armchair athlete today but a man who continues to practice precisely what he preaches. One recent year, while competing in the 26.2-mile New York City Marathon, I noticed him bobbing along in a flock of runners just ahead of me. Accelerating, I caught up with him, muttered a panting, perfunctory greeting, and tried to pass. Recognizing me, he made his move. The last I saw of him he was striding away into the distance, going strong.

JAMES F. FIXX

Preface

This book provides you with the simple basics for being physically fit. Regardless of your age or present state of fitness, you will find within these pages all the information you want or need to help you begin and maintain a program of healthy and enjoyable exercise.

Not only will you find easy to follow charts for walking, running, swimming, cycling, and many more healthy exercise activities, you will also find the latest information on why such exercise is good for you and how an active lifestyle will improve your health and well-being. You will learn the important particulars about being properly tested. Exercise charts that have been used in the Ball State Adult Fitness Program over the years are provided. These charts are included for you to follow at a reasonable and safe intensity — an effort level that helps you reap the benefits of becoming physically fit.

This book represents a sifting of the knowledge and experience I have acquired leading exercise programs for more than two decades. The simplicity of this book may surprise you. Wayne Anderson and I have assembled in this book, as concisely and clearly as possible, what you must know and do to develop a solid foundation of physical fitness. All the "flab" has been carefully edited out.

Instead of being enrolled in our adult physical fitness program, you are reading this book. That puts me at a disadvantage in trying to help you to become physically fit. We all know that teaching by the printed page is not easy. The most effective instruction calls for personal attention. But since this is not possible, I'm confident that the information on the pages that follow will bring you as close as any absentee can get to actually enrolling in our program.

The uniqueness of this book is that there are no gimmicks. It requires intelligent study and a willingness to read and follow the instructions and suggestions set forth for you. If you are unwilling to commit yourself to this, then call it off right now. On the other hand, if you want results, this book can help you.

Bud Getchell

Acknowledgements

Sincere thanks are due to many people who have directly or indirectly influenced the information found within this book. I am indebted to former professors, especially Dr. Thomas K. Cureton, Jr., who provided the initial spark for me while I was a Ph. D. student of the fascinating study of physical fitness at the University of Illinois.

Thanks must also go to my friends of expertise in sports medicine research who have supplemented the factual knowledge in this book and who are dedicated to seeking the "truth" about exercise training. I am most appreciative to the graduate students who have ably assisted me in exercise testing and leadership in recent years, and especially Nancy Nienaber for her contributions to the preliminary development of this manuscript. My sincere thanks to Sharon Ward, my secretary, for her efficient typing of the final drafts and for her able assistance throughout the project.

I am also grateful to the many students and older adults who have taken part in our Ball State University Physical Fitness Programs over the years. Their participation has provided me with insight into the practical applications of exercise principles. My sincere thanks must go to the people who allowed me to tell their stories in order to help others realize that exercise can be a positive force in living a full life.

A Note From Wayne Anderson

Before I met Bud Getchell I wasn't much aware or concerned about what I was physically doing to my body. I was overweight, smoked, and had high blood pressure, yet considered myself athletic because I played tennis on weekends. When we met in 1975 and started working on his college textbook, he considered me a challenge to his principles and techniques for getting someone who was out of control back into shape. I didn't make it easy for him. My job was to make his textbook a success, and its success didn't depend on my believing and following what was in it.

Eventually I gave in to Bud's friendly persuasion and started my own physical fitness program. That wasn't easy for me. I came up with numerous excuses for not putting on those shoes and hitting the pavement, for not swimming laps in the pool, for not working out on my exercise bike. Finally I realized I had to make a commitment to give his techniques a chance. They worked! Soon I began to see the results and felt good about what I was accomplishing. I was exercising because I wanted to, not because I was afraid he might call and ask how I was doing. I learned that exercising could become a part of my lifestyle and not interfere with my other daily activities.

Although I am the coauthor of this book, I am also one of those for whom it was written. Even though I exercise regularly, there's still room for improvement! Helping Bud write this new book has been more fun for me than working on the college textbook. Now I know that the guidelines presented actually work!

There are numerous books on how to get and stay physically fit, but none are as simple and easy to follow as this one. And none have Bud's friendly persuasion nudging you through the pages and into action. Since you care enough about yourself to read this book, why not go a step further and give Bud's guidelines and techniques a chance? They work!

How To Use This Book

1. *Start at the beginning of this book* and work progressively through Chapters 1 to 6. This will assure you of the basic philosophy and knowledge needed to use the rest of the book effectively. Even if you have a general knowledge of exercise and physical fitness training, it won't hurt to review the fundamentals.

2. *Learn the basics about your body.* The underlying philosophy of this book is that understanding how your body works both at rest and during exercise can help you to establish healthy exercise habits. This book includes enough elementary physiology to explain how your body responds to exercise and to establish the rationale for an effective program of exercise.

3. *Follow the recommendations for evaluating your current level of physical fitness* provided in Chapter 5. For those who are unable to undergo a comprehensive evaluation that includes an exercise tolerance test, alternative self-tests are recommended.

4. *Start your fitness exercise program at the proper place on the charts* given in Chapters 8 through 12. Don't try to make up in a few days what you have lost over the years. The charts for walking, running, cycling, swimming, and other alternatives provide clear instructions so that you will not fall into the most prevalent trap of fitness seekers: doing too much, too soon.

5. *Use this book with friends.* Participating with your spouse, family, or friends is an added bonus, whether you're beginning or maintaining an exercise program. The information in this book can be more easily learned if you can openly discuss some of the content with others.

6. *Make it your responsibility to be physically fit!* The responsibility for the content of these pages is ours; the responsibility for being fit is ultimately yours. We are confident that the information provided is all you need for properly starting and maintaining a beneficial exercise program. Our goal is showing you how. Your goal is being physically fit. GOOD LUCK!

chapter one

Becoming Physically Fit

This book is concerned with the human body — your body. Its purpose is to help you reap the joys of living at your fullest physical potential. There isn't any magic to becoming physically fit. It requires a commitment of a small portion of your time and some physical effort. This adjustment in your lifestyle in order to tune up your body and keep it running at peak efficiency is an investment that will pay you dividends over and over. Not only will you improve you physiological functions, you will enrich your psychological outlook on life. Properly performed exercises on a regular basis can enhance your physique, make you stronger, bring about a greater energy capacity, and help you become more confident and self-reliant Those who have followed the programs in this book have found being physically fit to be an invigorating and restorating experience.

The Need for Exercise

Fortunately, regular exercise has been recognized as necessary for personal health and well-being. However, many people are still reluctant to get involved in a lifestyle that includes exercise.

Some people still believe that we need less exercise as we grow older. In other words, as we get older, we are supposed to slow down and grow old gracefully. No! Our bodies were not made to be inactive. Our bodies were made to be used. The heart, lungs, blood vessels, bones, and muscles function better when stimulated regularly with proper exercise. When the body is not stimulated regularly, its functional capacities tend to decline, especially as we get older. Research indicates that this physiological decline can be slowed considerably with proper adherence to a sound exercise program.

As you know, our modern lifestyle fosters unfitness. Many

1

technological advances are intended to eliminate physical exertion from everyday activities. We have become accustomed to riding, sitting, and watching. After a bustling day at jobs that most likely involve little physical activity, we come home to sit in front of a TV to relax.

Television influences us in ways that may not be best for our health and well-being. According to this "electronic authority," we can buy a cure for every ailment. It preaches instant relief from headaches, tension, constipation, bad breath, insomnia, colds, aching joints, and upset stomachs. It perpetuates poor nutritional habits with constant messages that soft drinks, munchies, and fast foods are the American Way. It advertises the conveniences of owning every conceivable human energy-saving device. If we allow it, we could be conditioned into an almost effortless existence.

Besides this conditioning to do only what feels comfortable, we daily face a competitive society full of pressing domestic problems, business obligations, and deadline tensions. Such stresses involve physiological systems of the body and can damage our health.

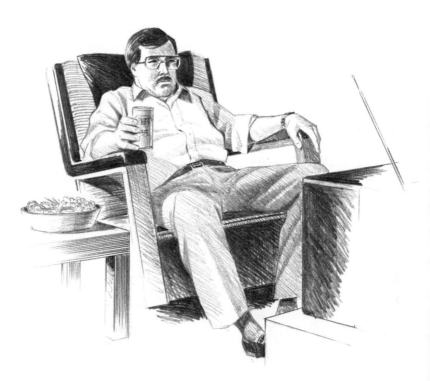

It's common for people to consider themselves healthy and physically fit if they are not actually suffering from an illness. But mere absence of illness doesn't mean we have good health and fitness. An inactive lifestyle causes unfavorable physiological changes. Muscles lose strength, body fat accumulates, the ability to keep up our everyday activities is lessened, the heart weakens, and the blood vessels thicken. Many of these changes go undetected. We tend to accept the resulting ailments as signs of aging — not the lack of physical activity.

Some people feel that their daily work provides them with enough exercise for their health and well-being. Running up and down stairs or standing all day at a job is physical exertion, of course, but such limited activities do not suffice for maintaining fitness. If normal, day-to-day activities leave you fatigued, then you need the increased energy and vitality that comes from regular physical exertion. The simple fact is *you must use energy to gain energy.* In other words, regular stimulation of the total body through vigorous exercise produces increased strength and endurance and many other characteristics that come with good health. These conditions can never be acquired by sitting at a desk all day, watching television, cleaning house, riding escalators and lawnmowers, or driving the car two blocks to pick up the kids.

Today, many people are on a renewed quest for sound health, fitness, and a quality lifestyle. One of the most visible signs of this trend is the emerging conviction among many that regular vigorous exercise can be a key to good health. With inactivity recognized as a menace to physiological well-being, some authorities suggest that exercise may be the cheapest preventive medicine in the world.

Exercise is not a panacea. But it is clear that, just as we need food, rest, and sleep, we need regular vigorous exertion to maintain our physical capabilities. I firmly believe that exercising regularly is the most sensible approach to establishing a lifestyle that will enable you to live at your fullest physical potential. Regular exercise may be the missing link in your quest for good health and total living.

What Does It Mean To Be Physically Fit?

Being physically fit means having your heart, blood vessels, lungs, and muscles functioning at peak efficiency. Peak or optimal efficiency means the high level of health we need for taking part in daily tasks and recreation with enthusiasm and pleasure. Being physically fit makes possible a lifestyle that inactive and unfit people cannot enjoy.

The four basic qualities of a physically fit body are strength, muscular endurance, flexibility, and cardiorespiratory endurance. A fifth quality is often added — neuromuscular skill, the general athletic skill reflected in the ability of your muscles to function harmoniously and efficiently. We see this quality in the flawless performance of skilled athletes. But although it's a desirable attribute, neuromuscular skill is not as essential as the other four qualities of a physically fit body.

Strength, probably the most familiar component of fitness, is the capacity of a muscle to exert or resist force. Strength training results in some enlargement of the muscle fibers and a relative increase in one's ability to apply force.

Strength is fundamental to all sports and many everyday activities. A lack of reasonable strength obviously contributes to poor performance. Strength is often lacking in the upper arms and shoulder regions, especially in women. This lack of strength not only impairs one's ability to swing a golf club or strike a tennis ball, but it can affect your ability to mow the lawn or do housework and related chores. A lack of strength is a major factor in the cause of back pain in many adults.

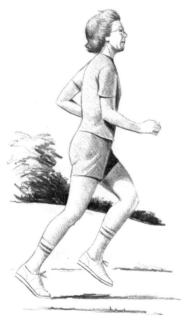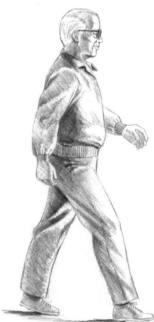

Muscular endurance is often incorrectly used to mean strength. It is the capacity of a muscle or a group of muscles to sustain repeated contractions. It also refers to the ability of a muscle to hold a fixed or static contraction over an extended period of time. In other words, it is the ability to apply strength and sustain it. Your ability to do sit-ups and pull-ups or to hang from a horizontal bar is a sign of muscular endurance. The capacity to perform activities around the home — shoveling snow, raking leaves, washing windows, painting, and cleaning house — all require some degree of prolonged muscular exertion.

Flexibility is the ability to use a muscle throughout its maximum range of motion. It is within your ability to move, bend, stretch, and twist your joints easily. Maintenance of good mobility at the major joints of the body provides good protection to muscles when subjected to physical exertion. Inflexible joints and muscles limit movement. The need for flexibility varies with your specific activities. Household tasks, outdoor gardening, and yard care require some degree of elasticity of the major muscle groups. Participation in most recreational sports and physical fitness activities requires a full range of muscle movement. Flexibility is the basis for gracefully coordinated movements.

Probably the most misunderstood component of fitness is *cardiorespiratory endurance*. Although the three physical fitness attributes just described are important, they are most effective when linked to the strength of the heart and lungs. Your life depends on the capacity of your heart, blood vessels, and lungs to deliver nutrients and oxygen to your body tissues, and to remove wastes. The function of this system is improved through vigorous endurance-type exercise. Many fail to see the need for developing this component of good health. They perceive the ability to perform prolonged periods of rhythmic exercise (such as walking, running, cycling, or swimming) as senseless. But exercise physiologists and medical researchers tell us that cardiorespiratory endurance is the *most* important quality of a physically fit body.

How Does Exercise Help *You* Become Physically Fit?

It is a physiological fact that the human organism needs stimulating exercise. When your total body is subjected to regular activity that involves vigorous stress of the heart, lungs, and muscles, the general efficiency of your physiological functions improves. When you are fit, your body will more easily adjust to increased physical demands. A physically fit heart beats at a lower rate and pumps more blood per beat at rest. As a result, your capacity to use oxygen increases, giving you more energy to enjoy life. Although regular exercise is not a cure-all, it is a sound means for achieving and maintaining a physically fit body. Being fit gives you the ability to do more and feel better when doing it. Getting more out of life is the reward of being fit. But can *you* experience this? Can exercise help *you*? Will being physically fit help keep *you* healthy? I am convinced of the health benefits of regular physical exercise, but I would be irresponsible if I answered these questions with an emphatic yes. The Ball State Fitness Program has helped many people, and if you follow the guidelines in this book, I think I can help you.

As you read through this book, you will gain information that can help you establish and reach a reasonably safe and attainable goal of physical fitness. Roughly, this goal is to be able to sustain an endurance-type activity at an effort level of 75% of your maximal capacity for a minimum of 30 minutes, four times a week. Most likely you won't attain this goal within the first few weeks of training. Therefore, I have provided exercise charts in a step-by-step format. Following the steps as presented will make it easier to exercise regularly within your capabilities and eventually become physically fit.

Making the Commitment

If you are determined to become physically fit, you need to accept this idea: *Exercising on a regular basis is a desirable behavior.* Therefore, you must structure your daily activities to achieve this desirable behavior. I want you to not only *think* fitness and health, I want you to *practice* fitness and health.

Whatever your reason for starting an exercise program, you must make a firm pledge to stay with it. When people start our program at Ball State, we always stress the importance of their personal commitment to attend the sessions regularly. If they can keep their commitment during the early weeks of the program, they will be well on their way to a lifetime of enjoyable and beneficial activity. As a general rule, it takes at least three to four months for most people to fully appreciate the pleasures of stimulating exercise. Therefore, you must stay with it long enough to realize the rewards. When you reach this point, you will likely be working out not because you *have to,* but because you *want to.*

You may wonder if you can handle such a commitment. The answer is *yes!* Daily living always takes some planning and discipline. Reporting to work, keeping business and social appointments, and meeting deadlines are already essential parts of our demanding lifestyles. Getting and keeping physically fit can become another commitment that we have built into our lives. It all comes back to the question of our priorities. Living at optimal physiological health has to be a top priority. If it is, then it warrants the investment of a reasonable amount of our time and effort.

There are 168 hours in a week. All we need is about four 30-minute workouts of sustained exercise per week to attain and maintain a reasonable fitness level. That's only two hours a week! A small investment of time and effort for such a large and beneficial return!

Getting Started

Keep two things in mind as you begin your exercise program: First, you can never begin too low (in the exercise charts), and the steps you take can never be too small. In other words, proceed carefully and don't be in a hurry. Injuries and discouragement result when you try to make up in a few weeks what you lost over many years of sedentary living.

Second, don't try to change everything at once. A regular exercise program usually provides an incentive to change such debilitating habits as smoking and overeating. But first, start getting into shape, Then you can more effectively tackle the problems of smoking and weight control. To enter an exercise program while cutting down on cigarettes and maintaining a strict, low-calorie diet is usually inviting failure. It takes an unusual person to make all these adjustments at once. Take one step at a time. The first step is to become active. Make activity and physical fitness your top priority. As you progress and your body becomes more attuned to exercise, then consider making gradual changes in your smoking and eating habits.

Staying With It

Once you've started an exercise program, you will occasionally confront stumbling blocks or obstacles to staying with it. Lack of time, illness (not necessarily your own), family obligations, just plain laziness (we all experience this), bad weather, and various types of injuries, just to name a few, can easily side track a well-intentioned fitness endeavor. Such conflicts can be disconcerting and, for some people, reason enough to quit. Let me suggest some ways to overcome these obstacles.

Finding time is the most difficult problem for many people. But as Jim Fixx, author of *The Complete Book of Running,* says, "Time isn't hard to find if you know where to look for it." He recommends that you honestly appraise your day, realizing that some sacrifices may be necessary. We have found (through trial and error) that early morning is the best time for our exercise program at Ball State University. This may not be the best time for you, but our participants have fewer business conflicts and interruptions at that time of day. Take a good look at your day's activities and find the time that's best for your schedule.

It's best to choose *a specific time* for your regular workout. Our experiences have shown that setting aside a specific time of the day to exercise will increase your chances of working out on a regular basis. At times, due to other obligations, you might have to change the time of your workout. However, setting a specific time for exercise lessens the chance that you will put it off. It's easy to say, "I'll do it tonight," and when evening comes, "I'll do it in the morning." Set a definite time that's best for you and stick to it.

Another tactic to keep you on a regular schedule is to work out with your spouse or a friend. Having to meet someone or picking someone up and driving to an exercise area together works for many people. Working out with friends can provide an incentive to keep you going. Group programs found at many YW/YMCAs, Jewish Community Centers, or private fitness centers provide an opportunity to meet and enjoy the company of others.

It also helps to keep a record of your workouts. This provides a progress report of your fitness program. Such a record is most helpful during the early weeks of training. It actually becomes fun to note such items as your time, distance covered, and how you feel after the workout.

A well-planned exercise workout strengthens your chances for improvement. However, don't expect to see instant improvement or each workout to result in progress. Successes and improvements in physical fitness come in spurts. Every day will not be a glorious one. Each workout will not result in euphoria. You will have some bad days. The progressive workout charts presented later in this book are planned to help you through good days and bad days. Each step on these charts is designed so that you can complete it without becoming overly fatigued and still provide the necessary stimulation to your heart, lungs, and muscles.

You may feel some discomfort when you exercise. This feeling will vary from day to day and from person to person. The important point to remember is that if you are quite uncomfortable or fatigued an hour after a workout, you are probably overdoing it. Therefore, you need to make some adjustment in your next workout. My aim is to show you how to keep your workouts reasonably comfortable and to avoid unnecessary fatigue.

The strongest reinforcement for staying with a regular exercise program is simply how you feel. After a few weeks you will feel stronger, more alert, and more relaxed than you did when you began. One of the main reasons people stay with an exercise program is that they really do feel better. Although feeling good is reason enough for exercise, taking off fat and maintaining a stronger heart and circulatory system are the bonuses of this more active lifestyle.

Keeping in shape will always take effort. But the rewards are well worth the effort. As you progress, you will be getting your body in shape and establishing habits that will become important aspects of your daily living. As you adjust to a more physical lifestyle, you will begin to enjoy the full benefits of exercise. Unfortunately, some people have not had the fortitude to reach this rewarding stage. It can be done if you make an effort to stay with your regular workouts. You can do it.!

Summary

Being physically fit means having a body that can function at its optimal efficiency. Being physically fit provides the robust health and the available excess energy needed to fully appreciate the joys of life. Put simply, being physically fit means doing more with quality!

This book provides sound guidelines for establishing an exercise program that cannot fail. But success in this program depends on your commitment. All the information about exercise in this book isn't going to help you unless you make the decision to start and stay with it. You can do it! You can become physically fit!

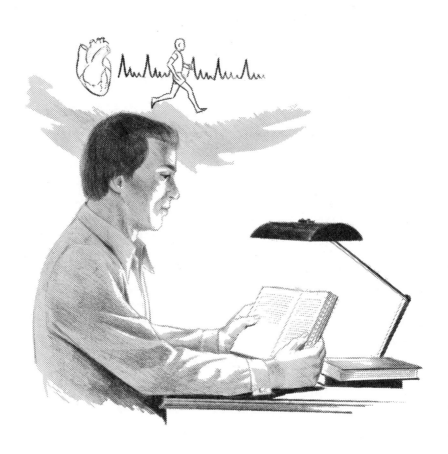

chapter two

Understanding How the Body Responds to Exercise

To be successful in your commitment to set up a lifelong fitness program you should have a clear understanding of how your body functions, how it responds to exercise, and how exercise improves it. Many people quit exercise programs or never get started because they lack such basic understanding of the body and why it needs the stimulus of regular exercise. We have found that understanding helps create a positive attitude toward physical fitness training and reinforces the commitment to stay with it. The purpose of this and the next chapter is to provide an overview of how your body functions, responds to exercise, and how it becomes stronger and more efficient with proper exercise.

The Basic Unit of the Body

The smallest structural and functional unit of the body is the *cell*. Cells are found in countless sizes and shapes. Most cells are so small that they can be seen only with the aid of high-powered microscopes; the human egg cell can be seen by the unaided eye. Protoplasm, the jellylike material that is the basic substance of all cells, is the medium in which complex biochemical tasks are continually carried out.

Groups of cells that perform a similar function form a *tissue*. Combinations of different kinds of tissue form an *organ*. And groups of organs form a unit of organization called an organ *system*. For example, various kinds of tissue, such as nerves, muscles, and connective tissue, are found in the heart — an organ. The heart, in

11

turn, is part of the circulatory system. Muscle tissues that attach to bones and span joints make up the skeletal muscular system. This system gives the body and its parts the ability to move. The nervous systems and endocrine systems control the functioning of the body. Nerves conduct impulses throughout the body and control muscle movement and other vital functions. Hormones, the substances secreted by the endocrine glands, serve as chemical messengers to help control the body's activities.

Muscle

A skeletal muscle is composed of groups of hairlike fibers that join into a tendon at each end. Each fiber is a cell in itself and can change its length when nerve impulses stimulate it.

The energy for movement of working muscles comes from the oxygen and nutrients that are supplied to the cells by the heart, lungs, and blood vessels. These same organs are responsible for removal of waste products. The physical fitness of a muscle can be understood as its capacity to use energy, to contract and cause movement.

All cells need energy to function. The nutrients from the food we eat and the oxygen in our bloodstream are utilized within the muscle cell in a series of chemical reactions to form ATP (adenosine triphosphate). An energy rich substance, ATP is found in every cell of the body and is necessary for contracting muscles, conducting nerve impulses, and performing other cell processes that require energy. Once the ATP is used, it must be restored. Therefore, more food and oxygen are needed by the cells. At times, especially during short, exhaustive exercise, an ample supply of oxygen isn't available in the muscle. Therefore, other mechanisms are needed to rebuild the ATP immediately. One of these processes is the use of CP (creatine phosphate). However, in a few quick seconds the CP supply is exhausted.

Another source of quick energy when oxygen is lacking is glycogen (stored energy). The breakdown of glycogen produces lactic acid (waste) and extends the ability of the muscle to contract until an accumulation of this waste becomes so great that the contraction stops. These events are called the anaerobic (without oxygen) phase of muscle chemistry because no oxygen is required. The anaerobic phase can last for only a few minutes. For contractions to continue, oxygen is needed to burn the available food in order to restore the CP and ATP. During this aerobic (with oxygen) process, 18 times more energy is released than during the anaerobic phase. In most types of exercise, the anaerobic and aerobic processes usually take place simultaneously. However, when performing rhythmic endurance-type exercise, most of the energy needs are aerobically provided. Rhythmic endurance-type exercise refers to physical activities that can be carried out continuously and rhythmically, such as walking, running, swimming, and cycling. They are often referred to as aerobic exercises. These types of exercises will be dealt with extensively in this book.

Human muscle is composed of two types of fibers — slow-twitch and fast-twitch. The *slow-twitch fiber* has a higher overall capacity for aerobic energy production than the fast-twitch fibers. It is the slow-twitch fibers that are recruited for movement during an extended period of rhythmic endurance-type exercise. These fibers provide the major portion of energy as we walk, run, or cycle. They have an extensive capillary network and are more able to take up oxygen for the energy processes than fast-twitch fibers. Thus, slow-twitch fibers better adapt to physical fitness endurance training than fast-twitch fibers.

On the other hand, *fast-twitch fibers* are specially adapted to short explosive bursts of contraction. These fibers provide an immediate source of energy when we suddenly run for a bus or up a flight of stairs or rush to the net in a tennis match.

In summary, the interrelationship of the various mechanisms in the muscle and body as we exercise is quite phenomenal. To effectively train these processes to function at their best is what this book is about.

Blood

Blood is an aqueous medium composed of blood cells, food stuff, minerals, gases, and many other substances that are vital to the proper functioning of the body. For example, the blood transports food stuff and oxygen to the tissues for the energy process. From the tissues, blood carries away cellular waste products and distributes the heat generated from the activities of the cell. The warmed blood cools as it moves near the skin of the body. Approximately 45% of the blood volume is composed of red blood cells, white blood cells, and platelets. The remainder is a liquid called *plasma*. The red blood cells are composed of iron-protein molecules, called hemoglobin, that combine readily with óxygen and carbon dioxide. When the situation demands, the red blood cells will easily give up these molecules. Plasma is a complex liquid consisting of foodstuff, minerals, hormones, and chemical substances needed by the cells for coordinating and regulating cellular functions.

The elastic vessels that carry blood away from the heart to the many tissues of the body are called *arteries*. The vessels that return the blood to the heart from the tissues are the *veins*. In the circulatory system, the arteries carry oxygen and nutrients to the tissue cells of the body. These cells receive their fuel and oxygen through thin-walled structures called capillaries that are distributed throughout tissues of the body. Carbon dioxide and other end-products are picked up from the tissue cells and carried back to the heart.

The Heart

The heart beats constantly. It pumps blood throughout the body at approximately 72 beats per minute, or over 100,000 beats in 24 hours. It circulates at least 2,000 gallons of blood a day. This powerful muscular pump never stops working regardless of the level of activity. After

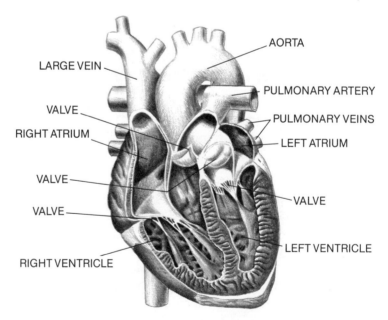

Figure 1. The heart.

climbing a flight of stairs, the skeletal muscles relax, but the heart keeps on beating.

The heart is composed of two upper chambers called *atria* and two lower chambers called *ventricles*. (See Figure 1.) The right atrium and the right ventricle are separated from their counterparts on the left side by a muscular wall. This separation allows the heart to work as two separate pumps (right and left). In addition, each atrium is connected to its corresponding ventricle by a one-way valve. The right atrium receives blood low in oxygen from the large veins, and pumps it through the right ventricle to the lungs. At the same time, the left atrium receives fresh, oxygenated blood from the lungs and pumps it out through the left ventricle into the *aorta,* the largest artery in the body, and ultimately to all tissues of the body.

Contrary to what you might expect, the blood passing through the heart does not nourish the heart muscle itself. Instead, arteries called *coronary arteries,* which branch off from the aorta, direct blood by way of capillaries to the cardiac (heart) muscle. (See Figure 2.) In this way each cardiac muscle fiber receives nourishment. The blood is then returned to the right atrium through the coronary sinus, a large vein formed by the coronary veins.

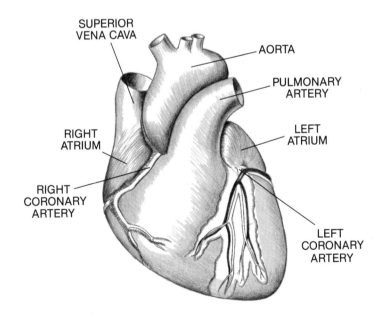

Figure 2. Heart with coronary arteries.

The Lungs

The lungs, located within the rib cage, are the organs that regulate the exchange of the air between blood and the external environment. Air enters the body by either the nose or mouth. It then passes into the throat, which is also a passageway for food. The throat branches into two tubes — the *esophagus,* through which food passes to the stomach, and the *trachea,* through which air passes to the lungs. The trachea extends downward toward the lungs. It divides into two branches, the *bronchial tubes,* one leading to each lung. Within each lung, each branch divides and subdivides through the entire organ. Eventually, this subdivision ends in tiny ducts (tubular passages) attached to an estimated one billion microscopic air sacs. These air sacs are clustered together, giving the lungs a spongy texture. Blood capillaries surround the air sacs.

When air is breathed into the lungs, the oxygen molecules pass through the walls of the air sacs into the capillaries. There they combine with molecules of hemoglobin, the protein-iron pigment in the red blood cells. From the lungs, this oxygenated blood returns to the heart, which pumps it to all parts of the body. Throughout the body, oxygen is picked up by the cells that need it, and the blood in turn picks up carbon dioxide and other waste products. This carbon dioxide is returned through the system of veins to the heart and then to the lungs where it is given up and eventually breathed out through the nose and mouth.

The Cardiorespiratory System

The heart, lungs, blood, and various muscle cells are interdependent parts making up the cardiorespiratory system. As noted previously, the maintenance of life depends on efficient operation of the body at the cellular level. Each cell needs a ready supply of oxygen and food, while carbon dioxide and other waste products must be carried away from it. Adequate functioning of the *cardiovascular* (heart and blood vessels) and *respiratory* (lungs and air passages) systems is needed for these life sustaining services. The cardiovascular system keeps the blood circulating throughout the body. The respiratory system removes carbon dioxide and replaces it with fresh oxygen. Because of their dependence on each other, the two systems are often referred to jointly as the cardiorespiratory system. Healthy functioning of the cardiorespiratory system is of paramount importance.

The heart, lungs and muscles respond to exercise in a predictable manner. When we change from rest to vigorous activity, our heart rate, blood pressure, and lung function automatically adjust.

Heart Rate

The heart rate and the amount of blood pumped with each heart beat (stroke volume) vary with the changing needs of the body. At rest the heart pumps about five liters of blood per minute. A liter is the unit of volume in the metric system, equal to 1,000 milliliters, or 1.06 quarts. But the heart is capable of increasing this output to 15 to 25 liters per minute when the body is active.

Your resting (sitting) heart rate is influenced by your age, level of cardiorespiratory fitness, and environmental factors. It becomes progressively lower as your fitness status improves. Changes in temperature and altitude can also affect heart rate.

Resting heart rates vary from extremes of below 40 beats per minute in highly trained athletes to over 100 beats per minute in sedentary adults. Women tend to have higher sitting heart rates than men. Seventy-two beats per minute is the average for most adults. However, in older people, especially those who exercise on a regular basis, rates are sometimes between 50 to 60 beats per minutes or lower.

As you begin to exercise, your heart rate increases. During low levels of exercise that can be sustained over a period of time (such as walking) the elevated heart rate will level out at a constant rate (steady state). The increase in heart rate during exercise is directly proportional to the intensity of the exercise. In other words, as the workload increases, the heart rate increases to a similar degree.

An example of this is shown in Figure 3. Notice how the heart rate increases as the walking speed increases from 3.0 mph to a brisker pace of 3.5 mph (a 17-minute-per-mile speed). At the four-minute mark the heart rate of this 53-year-old-man was at 136 beats per minute. The man had been sedentary prior to this test. After four minutes of level walking, the incline of the treadmill (a motorized conveyer belt commonly used for testing fitness) was raised to 4% and every two minutes thereafter, increased 2%. Note how the heart rates increase according-

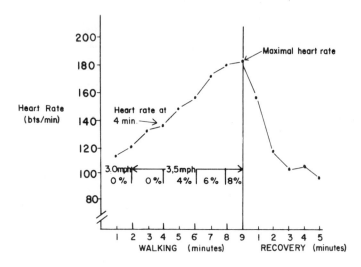

Figure 3. Heart rate responses to walking on a treadmill.

ly as the body responds to the increased demands of each grade of the walking task. This increase in heart rate is in direct proportion to the increase in workload, up to a limit. As his exercise workload becomes tougher, he eventually reaches the stage of the test where he had to stop (at 8% grade and at the 9-minute mark). At this point his heart rate of 183 beats per minute represents his highest attainable heart rate or maximal heart rate. In other words, when you perform strenuous exercise to a point of exhaustion, the heart rate at this point is your maximal or peak heart rate.

Maximal heart rates of 180 to 200 beats per minute are quite common. However, it is well documented that your maximal heart rate declines with age. It has little relationship to your state of fitness and can generally be estimated to be close to 220 minus your age. As you can see, applying this rule for estimating the 53-year-old man's maximal heart rate would grossly underestimate his actual maximal rate. Thus, when feasible, it is wise to be tested to determine your maximal heart rate. (Chapter 5 explains this in greater detail.) Knowing your maximal heart rate helps you determine your training or target heart rate, an important factor when determining how hard you should work out. (See Chapter 4.)

For any given heart rate, the heart with the largest capacity per beat (the largest stroke volume) will pump the most blood. That is, it has a higher cardiac output (pumping more blood per minute) for the same heart rate. *Stroke volume times heart rate equals cardiac output.* The larger the stroke volume, the greater the heart's ability to pump blood and the higher the level of performance.

Heart rate responses to standardized exercise tests (tests utilizing the same working rate) are convenient indicators of circulatory efficiency and fitness. Figure 4 shows the heart rate data for Jim, a man who started our program in 1973 when he was 57 years old. Jim's heart rate was monitored while he walked for nine minutes on a submaximal treadmill test. He was tested before beginning a run-walk exercise program and again after ten weeks of training four days a week. Jim was able to run a little over a mile without stopping when he was tested at the ten-week point. At this time his heart's response for the same walking task clearly shows a more efficient circulatory response. In other words, he improved. Notice that his heart rate at each minute of walking was decidedly lower throughout the submaximal walk than it was prior to training. Accordingly, his heart was pumping the same amount of blood more efficiently, with a lower heart rate and a relatively higher stroke volume. To further illustrate the effects of training on the heart, Jim was tested eight years later performing the same walking task. Jim, who runs four times a week and now averages three miles each workout,

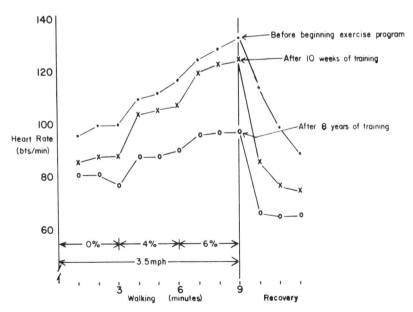

Figure 4. Heart rate changes due to training.

performed even more efficiently. Notice a lower heart rate throughout each minute of the walking test. At the last minute of exercise the graph clearly shows a drop in heart rate from 133 (beginning of program) to 124 (after ten weeks) to a much lower 97 after eight years of regular exercise.

A more rapid recovery of the heart rate after a workout also indicates cardiac efficiency. Again look at Figure 4 and notice how Jim's heart recovered faster after ten weeks and after eight years of training. In short, the physically fit person generally has a lower heart rate and a more rapid recovery time for any given exercise workload.

Blood Pressure

Blood pressure refers to the amount of pressure maintained in your arteries by the pumping action of your heart and the resistance of your blood vessels to blood flow. Blood pressure is generally recorded as two numbers. The higher number (*systolic* pressure) reflects the force that the blood exerts against the walls of the vessels as the heart contracts and ejects blood. The lower number (*diastolic* pressure) measures the reduced pressure in the arteries as the blood flows toward the veins and the heart relaxes and refills.

Systolic pressure in a normal, healthy individual while sitting is approximately 120 mmHg (millimeters of mercury pressure), and the diastolic pressure is around 80 mmHg. *Hypertension* means high arterial pressure, or simply "high blood pressure." A resting pressure of 140/90 or higher is generally considered high blood pressure.

For many who have an elevated blood pressure, the cause is unknown. However, we do know that high blood pressure places an abnormal strain on the heart and arteries. Also, it is well established that high blood pressure is a heart disease risk factor. Because of this, many doctors feel that even a mild case of high blood pressure is cause for concern and warrants attention.

Although blood pressure can be lowered through medication and diet, for many it can also be lowered through regular, vigorous exercise. Advances in pharmaceutical medicine have made it possible to reduce the dangers of elevated blood pressure through regular medication. But rhythmic endurance-type exercises such as running, swimming, cycling, and walking have also proved to be sound means for lowering the resting blood pressure and keeping it down. During

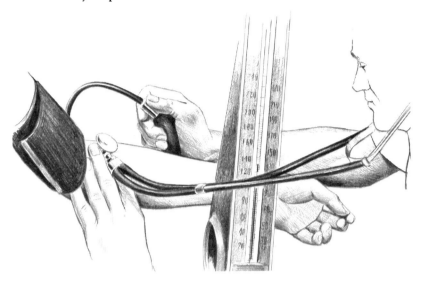

exercise, the systolic pressure increases, primarily because of increases in cardiac output. This rise in blood pressure is a normal response and is related to the intensity of the activities. Thus, heavier workloads produce higher systolic pressures. It is believed that this increase in pressure and the resulting dilation of the arteries while exercising tend to benefit the blood-flow mechanisms.

Lung Function

Physical exertion increases the need for oxygen in the cells. At rest the lungs breathe in about six to eight liters of air each minute, resulting in about a quarter of a liter of oxygen getting to the body's tissues. With even the mildest exertion, the lungs must breathe in more air. The amount of increase depends upon the intensity and the duration of the exertion. While walking, climbing stairs, running, or cycling, for instance, considerably more oxygen is needed, which causes breathing to increase rapidly in both depth (volume) and rate (breaths per minute). This increase may go as high as 60 to 100 liters of air per minute in the average sedentary adult and to over 150 liters of air per minute in a well-conditioned athlete. Thus the demand for more oxygen as the intensity of exercise is increased is met by an increased ventilation (breathing) of the lungs and blood flow (carrying oxygen.) The ability to improve the capacity of these physiological responses with vigorous exercise is the key factor in developing a healthy and fit body.

During exercise, an inability to get enough oxygen and the build-up of carbon dioxide, a waste product, hinders the ability of the muscles to contract, impairing movement. As previously noted, the oxygen requirement at the cellular level of the entire body ranges from a quarter of a liter at rest to a maximum of four liters or more at high levels of activity. But it is well known that the lungs always contain ample oxygen for the circulating blood to pick up as it passes through them. Furthermore, the oxygenated blood leaving the lungs and returning to the heart is almost always saturated with oxygen — that is, the blood is holding all the oxygen it can. The problem, therefore, is to get more blood to the active muscle tissue to meet the needs of exertion. These needs can be met by increasing the speed with which the blood goes through the cardiovascular system.

For example, if an activity requires three liters of oxygen a minute, but the heart can only pump enough blood to supply two liters of oxygen per minute, in a short time the build-up of metabolic wastes in the cells and the shortage of oxygen will reduce the capacity for movement. Eventually movement will have to stop. In short, your muscles are fatigued. If the heart was able to pump adequate blood to supply three liters of oxygen to the muscle tissues, then the activity could continue without fatigue occurring. How effectively your cardiorespiratory system responds in producing more energy for bodily functions depends in part on your physical fitness. From this example, you can easily recognize the importance of the heart's ability to pump large amounts of blood during exercise.

The ability of your heart to pump blood and of your muscle fibers to take up oxygen are the keys to successful muscular performance. The circulation and respiration systems limit your exercise performance to the degree that your heart, lungs, and blood vessels can function at their greatest potential. Unfortunately, many people, because of an inactive lifestyle, can't pump sufficient blood in time of stress. The feeling of being out of breath or exhausted during even mild exercise is not due to a shortage of oxygen in the lungs. Rather, it is due to an inability of the heart to pump sufficient blood to the muscle tissues, as well as an inability of the cells to take up adequate amounts of oxygen to meet the energy needs.

Aerobic Capacity (Maximal Oxygen Uptake)

As previously mentioned, the body is in constant need of oxygen. The ability of the body to utilize oxygen depends on the efficiency of the cardiorespiratory system. During vigorous activity, the exercising muscles use increased amounts of oxygen and produce corresponding amounts of carbon dioxide.

The largest amount of oxygen that you can consume per minute is called your *maximal oxygen uptake*. This maximal value, often referred to as *maximal aerobic capacity*, is a functional measure of physical fitness. The capacity to sustain effort over a prolonged period of time is limited by the ability to deliver oxygen to the active tissues. Theoretically, a higher oxygen uptake indicates an increased ability of the heart to pump blood, of the lungs to ventilate larger volumes of air, and of the muscle cells to take up oxygen and remove carbon dioxide. Therefore, maximal oxygen uptake is a measure of maximal cardiorespiratory function.

Not all of us can improve our maximal oxygen uptake to the same extent with similar types of training. It seems each of us has a certain potential for optimal development that has been genetically determined. In other words, the physical characteristics of our parents predisposes some of us to have more favorable adaptations to training than others. Regular vigorous exercise will produce a training effect that can increase your maximal aerobic capacity by as much as 20 to 30%. However, the precise amount of increase depends on your genetic endowment, your initial fitness level, and the intensity and duration of your exercise program.

Measuring Aerobic Capacity

By regulating the workload on a motor-driven treadmill (conveyor belt) with the speed and the angle of the incline progressively increased, your body's ability to use oxygen can be measured. To perform the test, one walks or runs on the belt, following a pattern of increasing workloads until exhaustion. A bicycle ergometer (stationary bike) is often used as an alternative when a treadmill is not available. With this device, precise settings of resistance can be set accurately at each stage of testing.

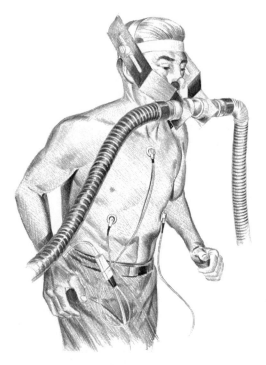

The volume of expired air is measured, and samples of this air are analyzed for their oxygen and carbon dioxide contents. Knowing the volume of air breathed and its oxygen and carbon dioxide contents, the amount of oxygen consumed by the subject can be calculated. By exercising subjects to their highest levels (when they can do no more), their aerobic capacity, or maximal oxygen uptake, can be determined. This universally accepted value represents not only a measure of the functional ability of the heart and lungs, it also measures the exercising muscles' capacity to extract and utilize the oxygen delivered to them by the blood. A more complete explanation of exercise tolerance testing will follow in Chapter 5.

Maximal oxygen uptake is usually expressed as the amount of oxygen (expressed in milliliters) that can be consumed for each kilogram of body weight (a kilogram equals 2.2 pounds and 1,000 ml equals one liter, or approximately one quart). The highest aerobic capacity ever recorded was measured in a male Scandinavian cross-country skier: 94 ml/kg·min. The highest female value, 74 ml/kg·min, also belonged to a Scandinavian cross-country skier. Champion marathoners have been found to have values of about 75 to

82 ml/kg·min. In 1978, Bill Rogers was tested at our Human Performance Laboratory at Ball State University about three weeks after he won the New York City Marathon. His value was a respectable 78.5 ml/kg·min. For comparison, we tested a group of runners (age 40 plus) who qualified for the Boston Marathon that previous spring. Their measured maximal oxygen uptakes (aerobic capacities) were between 58 and 62 ml/kg·min. As would be expected, they all finished the 26.2 miles distance an hour to an hour and one half behind Rogers.

Your oxygen uptake at rest (sitting) is about 0.25 liters per minute (often expressed at 3.5 ml/kg·min, or one MET). A MET is a term used universally by exercise leaders to represent the energy cost value at rest. During a vigorous exercise workout, it is possible for your oxygen uptake to increase to 8 to 12 times your resting value (8 to 12 METs). In fact, oxygen uptake values at "max" for fit people will range from 10 to 15 or more times their resting values. Keep in mind that your genetic make-up, sex, age, and state of physical fitness all help to determine your maximal aerobic capacity.

Sex Differences in Physiological Functions

To date, much of the data on the physiological responses of women to exercise have been generalized from the results of investigations on men. The standards of excellence in sports and physical fitness achievement have been based on male performances, and any achievement falling short of these standards has been interpreted as inferior. Whether or not the female's physiological responses are limited has not been determined. Research is beginning to suggest, however, that the way both sexes respond to vigorous physical activity is much more similar than different.

Our own studies of sedentary middle-age and older women and men have repeatedly shown that although the women had lower values for maximal oxygen uptake, their rate of improvement was similar to that of the men. Exercise heart rates also improved (that is, decreased) proportionately with those of the men. Loss of skinfold fat at selected sites was also comparable. Even though sexes differ in body size and structure their responses to vigorous exercise are essentially the same.

Many women fear that vigorous exercise will make them heavily muscled and unfeminine looking. There is no scientific evidence to substantiate this fear. Women normally have less muscle mass than men. However, the development of muscle mass is as varied among women as it is among men. Some women may be stronger and faster than some men. The inherent capacity for muscle development, however, is genetically determined by the sex hormone levels. The male hormone, testosterone, is responsible for muscle bulkiness in males. This hormone is present in women, but in amounts too low to have a substantial effect on muscle size. Dr. Joan Ullyot, a physician and running enthusiast, points out that compared to men, women in general have less muscle mass (23% compared to 40% muscle mass of a man's body), a lighter bone structure, and more body fat. Therefore, for people of the same height, a woman will usually weigh less than a man, and she will have less power to propel the same mass.

There have been recent claims that women naturally burn more fat as muscle fuel and perhaps may be more suited to endurance performance. To date, no laboratory evidence exists to substantiate this theory. However, we do know that endurance training does assist the working muscles for more efficient use of fat for energy. As for a woman's physiology having an advantage over a man's in long races and endurance-type events, there seems to be no scientific evidence for or against such a claim.

A woman cannot carry as much oxygen in her blood as a man, a factor that may limit her endurance. This is because women generally have fewer total red blood cells and about 15% less hemoglobin (the protein-iron molecule that carries oxygen in their blood) than men. The combination of a smaller muscle mass, fewer red blood cells, and lower hemoglobin means that women, in general, have less potential for endurance than men.

Specific Female Physiology

For years there have been many contradictory assertions about the relationship of physical activity to female physiological functions such as the menstruation cycle, pregnancy, and child-birth. The effects of physical conditioning on these functions are still not certain. Nevertheless, at the very least, regular, vigorous exercise appears to have no detrimental effect on women's physiology.

Menstruation

Today, vigorous exercise during the menstrual period is accepted more readily among medical practitioners and, more importantly, among women. Scientific evidence on the effects of exercise in a woman's body during this time of her cycle is limited, however. Recent articles summarizing the latest information clearly suggest that the normal routine of life should not be interrupted during menstruation. In fact, exercise has been cited as having great promise for preventing the monthly distress some women suffer. The bloatedness, tension, headaches, and loss of energy common during the premenstrual phase have been known to be helped with moderate exercise. Likewise, dysmenorrhea (painful cramps) can often be eased by moderate exercise such as walking and slow running.

The athletic performance of some women may suffer during premenstrual or early menstrual days. Simply worrying about the effect of menstruation might have a detrimental influence on performance. Nevertheless, women have won Olympic medals during every phase of their menstrual cycle.

As women increase their participation in vigorous endurance exercise (such as running and swimming), reports of deviations from the normal rhythmic pattern of the menstrual cycle have also increased. Amenorrhea (cessation of menstruation not due to pregnancy) is becoming widespread among female distance runners. Explanations for this exercise-produced amenorrhea are still speculative. Greatly reduced body fat, as well as the stress of intensive training, have been the two most common possibilities for this alteration in the menstrual cycle. One or two missed periods is not a major concern for a normal, healthy woman who is regularly engaging in vigorous exercise. Nevertheless, if this condition persists, a doctor should be consulted. In general, women with a high degree of physiological fitness appear not to be bothered as much by the most common gynecological problems as women who are unfit.

Fortunately, the greater freedom for women to be physically active has done much to change misconceptions and attitudes about menstruation. Since the menstrual period is a normal physiological function, a woman should be encouraged to continue her regular exercise habits during her period. As more and more women become involved in vigorous, rhythmic endurance-type exercise, new scientific findings will undoubtedly substantiate some of our recent opinions and personal insights about the positive benefits of exercise for women.

Pregnancy and Childbirth

Research also offers limited guidelines on exercise for pregnant women. Heavy training for athletic competition, especially during the final three months of pregnancy, has been frowned upon. However, when a woman has been physically active since before conception, continuing her exercise program during pregnancy seems permissable. The fetus is well cushioned, floating in a sack of fluid that acts as a shock absorber. Such activities as running, walking, and cycling cannot harm the baby. In contrast, engaging in springboard diving, gymnastics, judo, and similar activities are risky.

Most authorities recommend that a pregnant woman continue her normal physical fitness activities, though taking care not to become over fatigued. In fact, this is sound advice for anyone in a physical fitness training program, pregnant or not. There is no need to overdo it.

Beginning a vigorous program of physical conditioning at the onset of pregnancy, however, might be unwise. Crash exercise programs during pregnancy cannot substitute for long-term, regular physical conditioning. If you choose to begin a program during pregnancy, you should seek medical consultation and supervision from an authority on exercise.

Women who have athletic backgrounds or who are habitually active tend to have a smaller incidence of complications during pregnancy, as well as quicker and easier deliveries than those who are sedentary. Their cardiorespiratory system, muscle control, and abdominal muscles can speed labor for the simple reason that they can bear down during delivery.

Summary

The human body was made to be used. Understanding how the body responds to exercise and why it needs regular stimulation is important in helping you to set up a personal exercise program. I hope you now understand why the body improves with use and declines with disuse.

In this chapter only the fundamentals of exercise physiology have been presented. The next chapter provides you with more specific facts on how properly practiced programs of exercise can benefit you. Supportive data on how rhythmic endurance-type exercise improves the health of your heart, lungs, and vascular system are covered. Hopefully this understanding will provide the basis for not only understanding the chapters to follow but a foundation for a successful commitment to a lifelong fitness program.

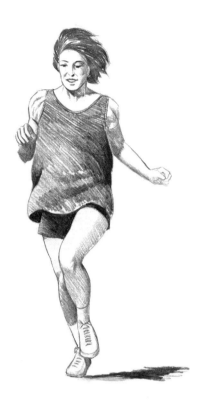

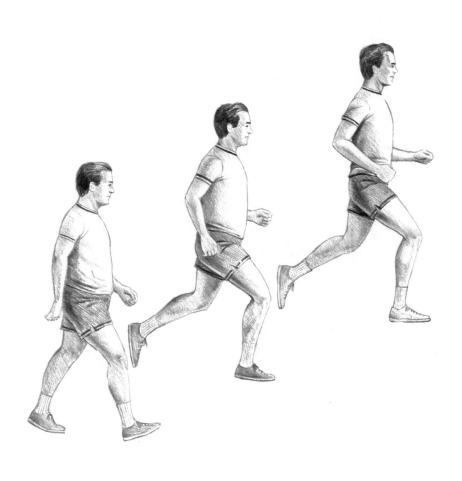

chapter three

The Benefits of Exercise

Much has been written proclaiming the benefits of exercise and of being fit. Unfortunately, many of the claims have gone too far and implied that any kind of exercise is good for you. Enthusiastic promoters often make statements that are not true or have not survived a rigorous scientific study. Everything from the tightening of gums to the restoration of a sexual life has been promised. This is not to say that such testimonies are false, but many statements are questionable because of improperly controlled research.

This chapter explains the beneficial effects of regular participation in various exercises so that you will know what they can and cannot do for you. I will tell you what we know to be the most reasonable results for the average person. Rhythmic endurance-type exercise practiced under certain conditions (that is, according to the guidelines in Chapter 4) can yield positive effects in a predictable manner. Under normal circumstances the body is more likely than not to benefit from endurance-type exercise. But the extent of the benefits varies from person to person.

In recent years much research on the effects of exercise training on the human body has been conducted in laboratories throughout the world. Unfortunately some of the results of these inquiries never reach the general public. And often research results are twisted, taken out of context, or unknowingly misinterpreted. Many of the promoters and manufacturers of the weight-training devices make claims that you can fully develop cardiorespiratory fitness by just using their equipment. Although many scientific studies have refuted such claims, these promoters artfully cite research, being careful not to say too much, but just enough to lead you to believe what they want you to believe.

To date, controlled laboratory studies have shown that exercise *is* good for the body and the mind, but that some forms of exercise are better than others. Therefore, it's important for you to select activities that are best for you and best for developing and maintaining cardio-respiratory fitness, and incorporate them into a reasonable and safe plan of exercise. The programs in this book are specifically designed to guide you through the early stages of getting in shape. These plans are based on the latest principles of exercise training, our own research, and valid scientific study conducted by responsible researchers throughout the world.

Walking, running, cycling, and swimming have been the most common exercises to be researched. How these activities can be performed to bring about optimal fitness has been the subject of many studies. Most studies dealing with cardiorespiratory fitness have employed training regimens that progressively increase the exercise workload as improvement occurs. They have been concerned with how the body adapts to varying intensities of exercise, within the tolerance level of the participants.

In Chapter 4 we will show you how to apply the basic information derived from controlled research studies that will help you plan for the conditioning needs of your heart, circulation, and muscles. With the application of these principles, whether you walk, run, swim, or cycle, you will be in a program that has been scientifically tested.

Some of the immediately noticeable effects of vigorous exercise are deep breathing, profuse sweating, and a rapid beating of the heart. These changes from rest occur whether you are in shape or not. If you continue to exercise vigorously on a regular basis, with sufficient overload and well within your tolerance level, favorable benefits will gradually occur.

Does Exercise Prevent Coronary Heart Disease?

Before we answer this question, let's review the causes of heart disease. The heart has to be a sturdy muscle in order to contract 100,000 times a day with enough force to pump blood through many miles of blood vessels. However, as mentioned in the previous chapter, the blood pumped through the heart does not nourish the heart itself. Instead, the heart muscle is supplied with blood through its own vessels, the coronary arteries. Symptoms of coronary heart disease occur when these arteries are impaired by a build-up of cholesterol and associated fatty substances on the inner portion of the artery wall. (See Figure 5.) These deposits cause a thickening of the inner walls and a serious nar-

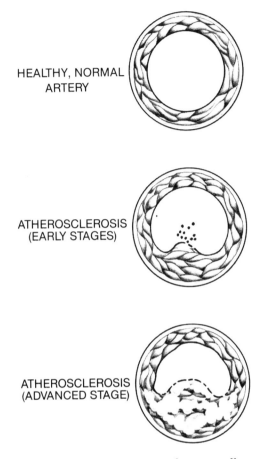

HEALTHY, NORMAL
ARTERY

ATHEROSCLEROSIS
(EARLY STAGES)

ATHEROSCLEROSIS
(ADVANCED STAGE)

Figure 5. Cross-sections of artery walls.

rowing of the blood vessels, a condition called *atherosclerosis*. The development of an obstruction of one or more arteries that supply oxygen to the heart muscle hinders blood flow, causing parts of the heart muscle to become impaired. Severe blockage may lead to *myocardial infarction,* the death of part of the heart muscle. This malfunction may seem sudden, but it has actually been building up to the crisis for years.

The best evidence of the early and gradual accumulation of fatty deposits in the body's arteries is a much-quoted study of 300 United States' soldiers killed in the Korean War. The subjects averaged only 22 years of age. When autopsied, 77% of them showed signs of diseases of the coronary arteries, from a slight thickening of the artery linings to complete occlusion (blockage) of one or more main artery branches.

Many of these young Americans had impaired circulation long before any symptoms would have appeared. But it's interesting that comparable studies of Korean soldiers killed alongside the Americans revealed no evidence of similar coronary damage. More recently, studies on Vietnam War casualties showed atherosclerosis in 45% of American soldiers. Studies in other countries (such as autopsies of accident victims) also show that early atherosclerosis is more common in young American men than in men elsewhere in the world.

This evidence suggests that coronary heart disease is not simply a disease of the elderly. Instead, this build-up of fatty substances in the arteries begins at an early age. Heart disease doesn't just happen overnight; it can begin in childhood and lead to a heart attack in the prime of life.

Despite recent declines, heart disease is the largest single cause of premature death in the United States. Over 150,000 Americans die prematurely (under 65) each year from heart attacks, and over 500,000 people suffer heart attacks that are not fatal each year. An additional 100,000 people each year have strokes (sudden or severe attacks caused by impaired blood flow to the brain), and 30,000 of these die. The mortality rates for men are several times higher than those for women. Nevertheless, American women lead those of all other countries in heart disease and stroke death rates.

Some experts call heart disease the "disease of prosperity"; others label it the "abuse of prosperity." The accomplishments of technology, automation, and science have raised our living standards, but the resulting soft living has made us vulnerable targets for heart disease. It is believed by many physicians and physiologists (myself included) that these premature heart attacks and strokes are preventable. The way we live can have an effect on the length of our lives.

Recently, medical and public attention has been directed to the prevention of coronary heart disease. In fact, this attention is one of the major reasons for the recent declines in death rates. Extensive medical research has identified certain so-called risk factors associated with increased cases of atherosclerosis. The greater the number of these coronary risk factors one has, the greater one's chance for heart disease and perhaps premature death. High blood pressure (hypertension), high levels of fats (cholesterol and triglycerides) in the blood, cigarette smoking, diabetes, obesity, certain emotional behaviors, and inactivity all have been linked to coronary heart disease. Other factors such as age, sex, race, and heredity are predetermined and cannot be readily controlled or remedied. But we can do something about diet, body fat, smoking, and exercise.

Although this book is primarily concerned with exercising properly, it is also concerned with other aspects of life that help enhance your health and well-being. Quite often, you will discover a need to change habits that are harmful. One of these harmful habits may be cigarette smoking.

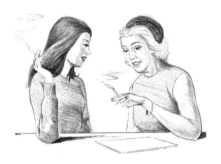

What About Smoking?

I would venture to predict that smokers who follow and adhere to the exercise guidelines in this book will eventually give up smoking. Three out of four smokers say they want to quit. Many have tried and failed. For many, cigarette smoking is an addiction and requires emotional and physical agonies to give it up. If you are a smoker, pursuing a disciplined exercise program may be the best answer to ridding yourself of the habit.

Confronting the evidence that cigarette smoking is harmful to your health is the first step. Permit me to quote the statement issued by the World Health Organization.

> "Smoking-related diseases are such important causes of disability and premature death in developed countries that the control of cigarette smoking could do more to improve health and prolong life in these countries than any single action in the whole field of preventive medicine."

According to cardiologist John W. Farquhar of the Stanford Medical School, cigarettes contribute much more to the incidence of heart attacks than they do to lung cancer. In fact, with other risk factors being equal, the average smoker is more than twice as likely to have a heart attack than the non-smoker. The Office of Smoking and Health in Washington, D.C., recently reported that a 42% drop in smoking has occurred among adult males during a recent 14-year span. But smoking among women, especially young women, has almost doubled during this same time period.

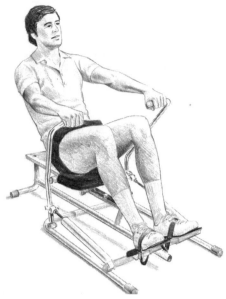

People who adhere to our Ball State program (as outlined in this book) quickly learn that rhythmic endurance-type exercise and smoking do not mix. When non-exercisers who smoke join our program they expect me to tell them to stop smoking. I don't. Instead, I want them to concentrate only on the beginning stages of getting in shape. Eventually, as they adjust to the early stages of the workouts, the positive effects of training are felt. Then they realize that smoking hinders their progress. This is not to imply that everyone who is in shape doesn't smoke.

A key reason to quit smoking is that the risk of coronary heart disease is decreased and after 10 years, the risk for premature heart disease is the same as for those who never smoked. Also, the risk of cancer is greatly reduced. Other possible benefits expressed by former smokers range from improved sleep to keener taste and smell.

The Case for Regular Exercise

Regular endurance-type exercise such as walking, running, cycling, and swimming can measurably improve the efficiency of the heart and circulation. The American Heart Association's committee on exercise advocates such physical activity "as an adjunct" to the control of blood pressure, blood fat levels, and obesity. They caution against the supposition that exercise alone will prevent heart disease. However, they

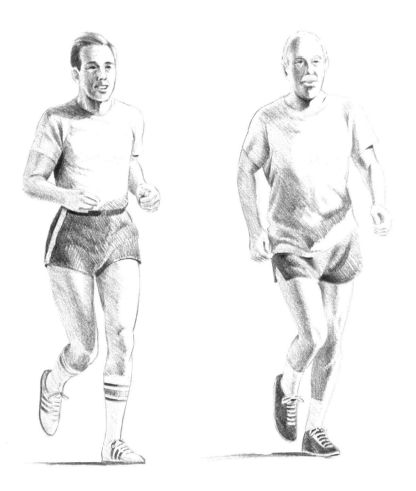

encourage exercise programs "tailored to the capacity and interest of the individual" for two reasons: they enrich the quality of life and, in combination with other measures (such as low-fat diets or eliminating smoking), help reduce coronary risk.

According to Dr. Samuel M. Fox, a leading cardiologist, the data relating to physical activity and heart disease *suggest,* but fall short of proving, that an increase in habitual physical activity prevents heart disease. Although we can not go so far as to say that regular endurance-type exercise prevents heart disease, there are predictable improvements to the cardiorespiratory system that are worthy of consideration.

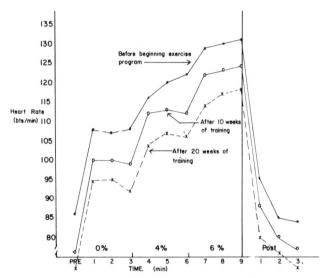

Figure 6. Heart rate changes due to training.

Cardiorespiratory Benefits

Improved Heart Function

After eight to ten weeks of vigorous endurance-type exercise performed on a regular basis (four times a week), your heart will begin to beat less, not only at rest but during everyday tasks. Your heart will be working more efficiently, pumping more blood with fewer strokes, and will recover more rapidly from bouts of exercise or any type of activity that stresses your body.

The cumulative effect of a drop in the number of heart beats over a 24-hour period is impressive. If your heart rate averages 80 beats a minute for a day (a common rate for unfit people), your heart will beat approximately 115,200 times a day. Let's say, as a result of exercise training, you reduce your average heart rate by ten beats (a common occurrence) for each minute of the day. You will save about 14,400 beats per day. In other words, by getting in shape with sustained endurance-type exercise your heart will beat less each day. In fact, many people in our program reduce their resting heart rates by as much as 20 or more beats per minute.

In addition, the increase in heart rate during exercise is less than before physical conditioning. Recall the example of Jim in the previous chapter and his reduced heart rate response to a standard walking task on a treadmill. Figure 6 presents similar information. It represents a group of eight previously non-exercising women who exercised using the guidelines and methods presented in this book. They walked for nine minutes at a moderate walking speed of three mph, or a 20-minute-mile pace. The treadmill was tilted after three minutes to a 4% grade and then after six minutes to a 6% grade. This test is often referred to as a submaximal test and most apparently healthy people (whether they exercise or not) should be able to complete it. As you look at the graph notice how the average heart rate for these women (average age 38) is lowered as they progress through 20 weeks of rhythmic endurance-type exercise. Throughout each minute of this moderate exercise task there was improvement. Notice that in the last (ninth) minute they averaged a heart rate of 131 at the start of the exercise program. Ten weeks later the ninth-minute heart rate was down to 124, and after 20 weeks of walking and running the heart rate was at 118 — a 13-beat reduction. This represents a simple illustration of the training effect on the heart. Therefore, proper exercise training can improve the pumping efficiency of your heart and strengthen it to perform more effectively both at rest and during all types of physical exertion.

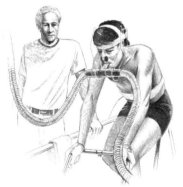

Improved Oxygen Uptake

As mentioned in the previous chapter, good cardiorespiratory function depends on the body's ability to utilize oxygen effectively. Our capacity to consume oxygen during exercise is enhanced by increases in cardiac output that result in greater volumes of blood (and therefore oxygen)

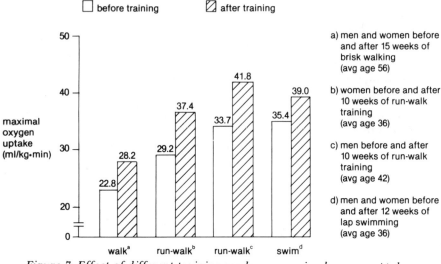

Figure 7. Effect of different training modes on maximal oxygen uptake

being delivered to the muscle cells. In addition, the muscle tissues develop mechanisms to use these greater volumes of oxygen. These adaptations, which readily result from rhythmic endurance-type training, are determined by measuring one's maximal oxygen uptake capacity. This measurement is widely accepted as the most representative sign of cardiorespiratory fitness. Because a larger person has more muscle mass and the capability to use more oxygen than the smaller person, aerobic capacity (maximal oxygen uptake) is expressed relative to body weight (ml/kg·min, or millileters of oxygen per kilogram of weight per minute). Young college-aged males and females range between values of 44 to 47 and 35 to 38 ml/kg·min, respectively. People who are older and people who lead a sedentary lifestyle tend to show lower values. In a 40-year-old man, aerobic capacity will drop to 30 to 34 ml/kg·min. Fortunately, exercise studies have shown that this decline in aerobic capacity as one ages can be slowed and even improved to the point where an older person's aerobic fitness can be higher than the average for younger people. Our studies clearly show that whether the exercise is walking, running, cycling, or swimming, one's cardiorespiratory (aerobic) capacity can be favorably improved. However, our experiences to date show that walking isn't likely to increase aerobic capacities to the levels associated with running. Figure 7 summarizes the effects of different modes of training on maximal oxygen uptake. Notice the levels of maximal oxygen uptake before training and the relative change over periods ranging from 10 to 15 weeks. Figure 8

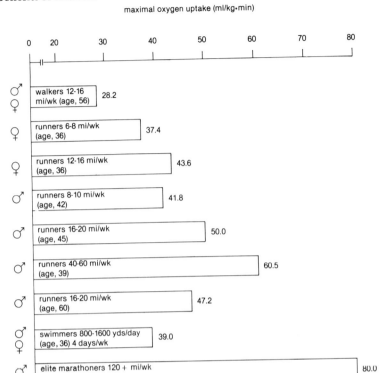

Figure 8. Maximal oxygen uptake of selected groups of active people.

shows results for people from our program after they have been in training for ten weeks or more. Some of these groups represent over a decade of training. Carefully study the average ages of these subgroups and the distance covered each week. You can readily see that the amount of mileage has a bearing on how high your maximal oxygen uptake can go. This graph points out some wide variations among people. However, recall that values close to or above 40 ml/kg·min represent a good level of cardiorespiratory fitness. Also included in this graph is a bar representing elite runners (mostly marathoners) to illustrate the top values. As you can see from this bar graph, improvements can be made over time and by progressing from walking to more vigorous activities like running or swimming.

Blood Pressure Changes

Several studies have indicated that active people tend to have lower resting blood pressures than most sedentary people. If your blood pressure is normal, vigorous endurance-type exercise has little if any effect on lowering your blood pressure. Some people who have high blood pressure, however, may see dramatic changes to a more normal level as the result of rhythmic endurance-type exercise training. If you have a weight problem, you are more likely to lower your blood pressure if you lose weight along with improving your fitness.

To say that exercise alone lowers blood pressure is still in question. For people who already have serious complications related to high blood pressure, the benefits of exercise for lowering blood pressure may be limited. The combination of an altered diet, medication, and exercise appears to be a promising approach to controlling this major risk factor of heart disease.

Blood Profile Benefits

The relationship between high blood *cholesterol* levels and heart disease has provoked much controversy for more than two decades. Cholesterol is produced in the liver. It is essential for cell structure and for the formation of various hormones, including sex hormones. Cholesterol and another fatty substance called *triglycerides* also make up the atherosclerotic deposits on the inner lining of the arteries that eventually may lead to heart disease. Medical researchers believe that cholesterol floating in the blood is in part the source of this continual accumulation.

The level of cholesterol in the blood can be measured. Any value above 250 milligrams (mg) per 100 milliliters (ml) of blood is considered dangerous. According to the American Heart Association, a person with a value of 250 or more mg per 100 ml, has about three times the risk of heart attack or stroke as a person with a cholesterol level below 200. Diets high in animal fat and cholesterol, and an inactive lifestyle are both related to high cholesterol in the blood. Adjusting the diet tends to lower cholesterol levels in some people. There is also evidence that physical fitness programs can reduce the level, but the role of exercise in controlling cholesterol is still not generally agreed upon.

The fat particles called triglycerides represent 95% of all fats stored in the body. In recent years the measurement of triglycerides in the blood has been used as an index of the number of fatty particles in the bloodstream. When more carbohydrates (sugar and starches) are eaten than are used for energy, the excess is turned into triglycerides (fat) transported in the blood and stored in fat cells situated throughout the body (such as on your abdomen, thighs, arms, and chin). These fats also seem to be related to atherosclerosis and, like cholesterol, can be lowered by weight loss through dieting and exercise. In fact, research experts have shown dramatic drops of triglyceride levels with exercise of the sort that increases cardiorespiratory fitness.

New findings from several heart disease studies suggest that it may be more important to know how cholesterol is carried in the bloodstream rather than just measuring the total amount present. Cholesterol is carried in the bloodstream by certain proteins, called lipoproteins because they carry a lipid (fat). Three types of lipoprotein are especially important to heart disease: high-density lipoprotein (HDL), low-density lipoprotein (LDL), and very-low-density lipoprotein (VLDL). The VLDLs transport triglycerides (which result from eating excess carbohydrates and calories) from the liver to the fat cells for storage throughout the body. The LDLs carry cholesterol from the liver to the cells of various tissues where it is used to make cell membranes and certain hormones.

For years the medical profession has known that the cholesterol being deposited in the arteries (atherosclerosis) is the cholesterol attached to the LDL. In contrast, the major function of HDLs is to clear unneeded cholesterol from the tissues and return it to the liver to be excreted. Although the role of HDLs is not clearly established, they are thought to prevent cholesterol from sticking to the inner walls of the arteries, thereby thwarting the process of atherosclerosis. In other words, evidence is accumulating that people with high levels of HDL-cholesterol in the blood tend to be relatively free of heart disease, whereas those with high LDL levels are more likely to suffer heart attacks. This has been verified by the often-quoted Framingham study (involving 5,000 men and women beginning in 1949 in Framingham, Massachusetts), which revealed that HDL-cholesterol is the most powerful single lipid predictor of coronary artery disease. In addition, recent reports (from Peter Wood of Stanford) indicate that middle-age runners tend to have higher levels of HDL (the "good" lipoprotein because it carries the excess cholesterol) than non-active people. There also appears to be less LDL among these runners. These preliminary studies *suggest* a case for vigorous exercise as a preventive measure for coronary heart disease.

At the Human Performance Laboratory at Ball State University we have been studying the effects of endurance training (walking and running) on HDL-cholesterol and triglycerides. At this point in our research it appears that although 10 to 20 weeks of endurance training does in fact increase one's fitness level, the favorable changes in the lipoprotein profile require a longer time period of training, perhaps a year or more. For instance, people who have been training for at least a year and running 25 miles or more a week have significantly better blood profiles than sedentary people who have been in endurance training for only a short period of time. We have observed for many years that it takes considerable training to lower total cholesterol and triglyceride levels. Nevertheless, it is quite common to see lower values, especially in triglycerides, in people who regularly run more than 20 miles a week.

Our research with swimmers and walkers shows that their training programs did not readily affect the lipid profile. We didn't begin to study lipoproteins until the fall of 1978. Perhaps as we follow these people over the years, and they increase the duration of their workouts, we will see a more favorable change in HDLs. Although research suggests that active people can raise their HDL levels and presumably move toward a more favorable risk category, it remains to be demonstrated how much activity and at what intensity these measures are affected. Weight loss and low-fat diet also seem to play an important part in bringing about favorable changes.

Exercising is no guarantee that you will live longer than your sedentary friends. However, if you exercise in an endurance-type activity that is vigorous and regular, you will probably live closer to your full genetic potential. A well-organized, vigorous physical fitness program should focus on adding more life to your years. But adding more years to your life may be the bonus for such a lifestyle.

Weight Control Benefits

Many people doubt that exercise is effective for weight loss. I firmly believe that, for most, being overweight is a problem of being inactive. Body weight can be controlled by engaging regularly in endurance-type exercise. As we grow older, our activity level tends to decrease while our appetite and eating habits do not. In fact, appetite may even increase with an inactive lifestyle.

Just dieting to control weight is seldom effective. Contrary to what some so-called weight control experts say, cutting back on calories does not complete the goal of a desired lean and healthy appearance. Exer-

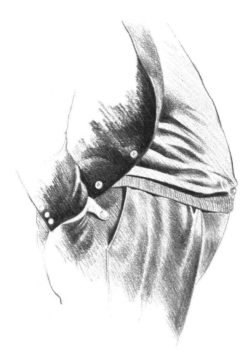

cise *must* be part of your weight control plan, or you will still look flabby and saggy.

Research shows that exercise or exercise with a modified diet is better for weight reduction than dieting alone, particularly in its effect on body composition and physical fitness. Although we have not studied people who only diet, we have observed changes in body composition of people who exercise. These changes reflect increases in lean muscle tissue as well as fat loss. However, during the early stages of training, as the muscle mass increases and fat burns off, the scale weight tends to remain the same, which, to the uninformed, becomes discouraging. In contrast, many special diets often result in rapid fluid loss and, in some cases, even loss of muscle tissue, leading to the false belief that fat has been lost.

Lean body tissue represents the bone-muscle-organ tissue of your body. Often called fat-free tissue, this part of your body gives it shape. Rhythmic endurance-type exercise such as brisk walking, running, swimming, and cycling builds up firm and supple muscles. As your muscles become stronger with exercise, they increase somewhat in size. However, these continuous and rhythmical activities will not make you bulky with muscles. And in women, this increase in muscle fiber thickness is not as great as in men. With the expected fat loss, your girths, if abnormally large to start with, will actually become smaller despite this muscle development. Our experiences (and the research reports of others) clearly suggest that exercise of the right kind is better than mere dieting, because it not only burns fat but tones and firms the muscles. And as a bonus, the exercise will improve the functioning of the heart, lungs, and circulatory system.

Exercise is the great variable in weight control. All of the chapters that follow provide sound principles for exercise that will help you realize the good feeling of controlling your weight and being fit. Chapter 14 is specifically concerned with helping you set up a plan for weight control.

Psychological Benefits

Among the most beneficial outcomes of vigorous activity are the psychological benefits. After working with hundreds of people of all ages and from all walks of life, I'm convinced that being fit is much more than having an efficiently working heart. Being fit gives an overall feeling of well-being. It bolsters your self-image and helps you to be more positive about yourself and those around you. Besides providing a diversion from the everyday work, engaging actively in sports and exercise provides an excellent relief and relaxtion for the mind.

Several recent studies support the belief that those who work out on a regular basis feel much better than those who do not. Such studies indicate that people who exercise regularly feel less tired, more disciplined, more relaxed, more productive at work, more satisfied with their looks, and more self-confident.

Doctor Ronald Lawrence, founder and former president of the American Medical Joggers Association, is convinced that vigorous exercise, in this case running, improves your total well-being. He feels that you sleep better, but need less sleep, your sex life is perked up, and you can better cope with stress and improve your work productivity. Whether the benefits are physical or mental, Dr. Lawrence keenly feels that vigorous activity strengthens the whole quality of life.

Doctor George Sheehan, cardiologist, runner, and author of several best-selling books on running, asserts that it is the psychology rather than the physiology of fitness that is important. According to Sheehan, "Play provides...physical grace, psychological ease, and personal

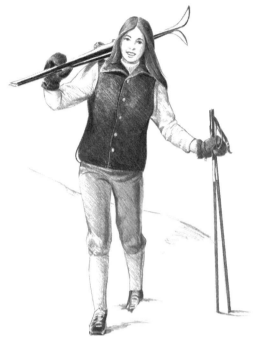

integrity. . . . One who plays is fulfilling himself and becoming the person he is." He recommends that you first become a good animal, know your body, and enjoy it. It is then that you discover play and fun. He believes that "exercise must be play or it will do little good." For Dr. Sheehan, running is an hour of play and enjoyment away from his daily routine. Although his words refer mainly to running, it is reasonable to assume that any endurance-type exercise or "play" can also provide a feeling of exhilaration. It can refresh the soul and provide a mental release. People who exercise regularly feel more alive.

Doctor Thaddeus Kostrubala, a San Diego psychiatrist, has had remarkable results treating his patients by having them run. This form of therapy has had profound mental effects on them. Depression was eased, medications abandoned, smoking and drinking reduced or eliminated, and overall well-being improved. Doctor Kostrubala suggests that vigorous activity such as running may cause some body chemistry reaction that helps to restore emotional stability.

Doctor Kenneth Cooper of the Aerobics Institute in Dallas feels strongly that people who are physically fit often tend to be psychologically fit. They exhibit a "fitness glow," and they feel better, look better, and have an improved self-image. Doctor Cooper suggests that when people become physically fit, they feel better because they are more relaxed, more in tune, more aware, and more perceptive.

Recently a study was reported in the *New England Medical Journal* that attempts to explain the "high" that runners and other exercisers often report. This research was conducted at the Massachusetts General Hospital in Boston. A small group of women who spent two months bicycling and jogging experienced dramatic increases in beta endorphin in their blood. Endorphin is an opium-like substance produced by the brain and pituitary gland that helps the body resist pain. The researchers attribute this increased release of these opium-like secretions as a possible explanation of "runners' high" — a condition that is similar to drug-induced euphoria.

Although hard evidence for such benefits is not yet available, the number of people who testify to such feelings is impressive. I constantly hear the same or similar testimonies from people in our program. To the non-exerciser, such declarations may be pure bunk. But maybe by now you are wondering why these committed exercisers are so verbal about the benefits they feel.

Summary

I hope you understand by now why your body needs a regular stimulus of aeorbic exercise. You should now be more aware of what changes to look forward to as you begin to follow the programs recommended in this book. The rest of this book provides the necessary know-how to help you realize the true benefits of exercise.

The next chapter explains the fundamentals of designing your own program and answers such questions as how hard, how long, and how often, you have to work out. It also presents the best activities for improving cardiorespiratory fitness.

I'm confident that if you carefully adhere to recommendations in the pages that follow you will discover new energies and the good feeling of being physically fit.

chapter four

Basic Guidelines for a Fitness Program

Many people are confused about the type and amount of exercise needed to become and stay fit. Some people who workout regularly started out improperly and found it a struggle. Fortunately, they survived the early rigors to become regular adherents. But for all those who made it, there are many more who didn't.

In my lectures throughout the country, the same basic questions are asked: How hard do I have to exercise? How far do I have to run? Do I have to run to be physically fit? How long do I need to work out? How often do I need to work out? What are the best activities for getting in shape? These are fundamental questions, and they need to be answered before starting or resuming a fitness program.

This chapter helps you answer these questions. The concepts and guideliness that are needed to set up a sound and reasonable program are provided. This information will help you determine for yourself what the best activities are and how hard you should work out to get the results you want.

The American College of Sports Medicine (ACSM) is a multi-disciplinary professional and scientific society dedicated to the generation and dissemination of knowledge concerning the motivation, responses, adaptations, and health aspects of persons engaged in exercise. It recently published a position paper based on the existing evidence from all over the world concerning exercise prescriptions for healthy adults. This paper summarized the most widely accepted guidelines for developing and maintaining cardiorespiratory fitness. The fitness training methods in this book are in accord with these guidelines.

The material in this chapter is not only the result of many years of working with all kinds of people, it also represents knowledge that has evolved from years of inquiry and experimentation by many sports medicine researchers. Such cooperative research efforts make it possible to organize principles of exercise training into a compact and easily understood format.

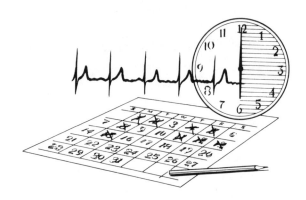

The Four Fundamental Factors

Although your fitness program should be tailored to your needs, the basic principles and guidelines for achieving a desired level of physical fitness are the same for all people. There are four essential ingredients for the development of a sound exercise program: (1) intensity — level of exertion; (2) duration — length of exertion; (3) frequency — number of workouts per week; and (4) mode — type of activity.

Intensity

To improve cardiorespiratory and muscular fitness, a vigorous *overload* is necessary in all conditioning and physical activity programs. This means a stimulation of the heart, lungs, and muscles with exercise of substantial effort but well within your capabilities. During exercise, the heart rate increases proportionately with the increase in energy requirement. In other words, as the exercise workload increases, the heart rate increases to a similar degree. For this reason, the exercise heart rate is used as a simple measure for estimating physiological stress on the body and is a standard means for determining exercise intensity levels.

To make appreciable gains in cardiorespiratory fitness, the heart rate during exercise (training heart rate) must be raised by approximately 75% of the difference between the sitting and maximal heart rates. This is referred to as your *75% heart rate reserve* and represents a safe and reasonable intensity for most participants. Working out at this heart rate level is a key factor in making significant progress in your fitness program.

How To Count Your Pulse

In order to control how hard you work out, you first need to learn how to count your pulse.

To determine your training or target heart rate, you must know your heart rate while sitting. And, to determine your exercise intensity, you need to know your heart rate immediately after exercise. Except in rare cases, the number of heartbeats each minute is equal to the number of pulse beats each minute. Therefore, your heart rate can be counted at any convenient pulse point.

Follow these steps to determine your pulse rate: First, get a stopwatch or a wristwatch with a second hand. Second, locate your most suitable pulse point. By placing the tips of the fingers on your chest, below and to the side of your left nipple, you can generally pick up your heartbeat. Or try your carotid artery, which is located just under your jaw bone on your neck slightly behind your Adam's apple. Taking your pulse on the inside of your wrist may be the best site. To do so, place the tips of two fingers immediately below the base of the thumb. Be sure to press lightly. (See Figure 9.) Third, when you feel your pulse, count the beats for 30 seconds. Then multiply your 30-second pulse rate by two to determine your pulse in beats per minute.

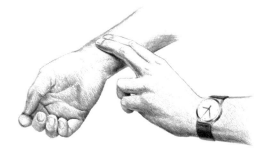

Figure 9. Counting your pulse.

It is easy to determine your heart rate at rest: just sit down in a chair and take your pulse. It is more difficult to take your pulse during exercise. For practical purposes it is assumed that the rate counted immediately following exercise is equivalent to the exercising rate. Immediately after exercise, the pulse rate declines rapidly, so it is important for you to learn to count your pulse as soon as possible (within a second or two after stopping). At this time, the pulse beats will be rapid and strong; hence, easier to locate. Find your pulse within a second or two of stopping exercise and count for ten seconds. Then multiply by six to get your heart rate for a minute. Remember your heart rate falls-off rapidly once you stop exercising so it is important to learn how to find and determine your pulse as soon as you stop exercising.

It will take a little practice before you can consistently obtain a reliable pulse rate. Through experimenting, you can find your most reliable pulse point. Taking your pulse rate immediately after vigorous bouts of exercise helps you monitor the intensity of your workout.

Determining Your Target Heart Rate

Determining your target or training heart rate is simple. Take the difference between your maximal and sitting rates, multiply it by 0.75, and add the result to your sitting rate. The maximal heart rate for most adults generally ranges between 170 and 190 beats per minute. This value represents your highest attainable heart rate. It has little relationship to your state of fitness. Although it is best determined by an exercise tolerance test (see Chapter 5), it can be estimated to be 220 minus your age. To estimate your training heart rate, use the formula below.

Formula for Estimating Your Target Heart Rate

220 − _____ = _____ Maximal Heart Rate
        Your Age

(_____) − (_____) = _____
  Maximal HR   Sitting HR   Heart Rate Reserve

(_____) × 0.75 = (_____) + (_____) = _____
  HR Reserve   Sitting HR   Target HR

Therefore, your target heart rate at 75% heart rate reserve = _____

Maximal heart rates vary between persons but decrease with age. For example, let's take a maximal heart rate of 180 (an estimate for a 40-year-old) and a sitting rate of 80. The difference is 100 beats. Seventy-five percent of 100 is 75 beats. Adding this figure to the resting rate of 80, we get a target heart rate of 155 beats (approximately 26 beats for ten seconds). This figure represents 75% HR reserve, the safe and effective training level for that person. Similar calculations for a maximal heart rate of 200 (a value for a young person) would result in a target heart rate (75% HR reserve) of 170.

When engaging in physical activity, you need to exercise close to your training heart rate to produce significant cardiorespiratory benefits. For most adults, this intensity means a target heart rate in the range of 140 to 160 beats per minute. For older adults, because of a decline in maximal heart rate with aging, a lower heart rate may represent an adequate training stimulus. A rate of 120 to 140 beats per minute may suffice. These intensities indicate safe levels of vigorous exercise for healthy people.

The table below presents a chart for converting ten-second pulse counts to beats per minute. For example, 26 beats for ten seconds is equivalent to an exercise heart rate of 156.

Conversion Table of Ten-Second Pulse Counts to Heart Rate

TEN-SECOND PULSE COUNTS	HEART RATE-BEATS/MINUTE
15	90
16	96
17	102
18	108
19	114
20	120
21	126
22	132
23	138
24	144
25	150
26	156
27	162
28	168
29	174
30	180

Duration

The duration of exercise is directly related to the intensity of the activity. Exertion at your target heart rate enables you to spread your workout session over a longer period of time than is allowed by a more intense level of exercise. Most research and our own experiences suggest that *an exercise session of 30 minutes* is sufficient to produce beneficial fitness changes. Thirty minutes seems to be the threshold for significant improvement even though there is some additional enhancement in cardiovascular functions from training sessions of up to an hour or more.

For a beginning program it is often unwise (and most unlikely) for you to be able to exercise continuously for 30 minutes or even reach a 75% level. Due to your present fitness level, your beginning workouts will most likely be limited to short periods of vigorous exercise alternated with more moderate levels of exercise such as walking. More on this later!

Frequency

Regular adherence to a vigorous exercise program is necessary if you are to reach and maintain an adequate level of physical fitness. Research indicates that training effects are both gained and lost rather quickly. Therefore you must work out regularly.

Surprisingly, we have found that daily activity, though desirable, is not necessary to improve one's cardiorespiratory fitness. Above-average physical fitness can be attained with *regular workouts four times per week*. Keep in mind, however, that improvements in many aspects of physical fitness continue over many months. It is wise to allow several of the initial weeks for adaptation. This recommendation is based on the assumption that your conditioning workouts will eventually be at your target heart rate intensity for at least 30 minutes. In our programs, adherence to such a vigorous physical fitness program has yielded physiological benefits for the participants.

Mode (Type of Activity)

Activities that are low in intensity and short in duration produce low levels of improvement. The relative values of various activities for improving physical fitness depend on the physiological intensity required. Golf, bowling, and softball, to name a few, do little to develop or maintain physical fitness. These activities are great fun, but they do not provide the necessary physiological stimulus for developing or maintaining fitness. However, *vigorous, continuous, and rhythmic activities* that involve the large muscle groups (such as brisk walking, running, cycling, and swimming) can be excellent for the development of the entire body. Such activities force the heart to beat at a rhythmic rate that is high enough to produce a training effect, challenging your cardiorespiratory system.

In general, activities that require short bursts of speed and quick movements do little to improve your cardiorespiratory system. For example, 30 to 60 minutes of racquetball or tennis, even four days a week, is not as good as rhythmic, endurance-type activities for substantial physical fitness. Obviously, the skill of the participant determines the training benefit of any sports activity. If you and your opponent have a reasonable amount of skill, you may be able to stay active enough to keep your heart rate elevated for conditioning purposes. However, a sustained workout for 30 minutes at your 75% HR reserve intensity four days a week, will produce greater cardiorespiratory fitness. You will be better prepared for your racquetball or tennis game. In other words, you get in shape to play your favorite sports rather than getting in shape by playing.

If you have been inactive, you should avoid highly competitive sports, which usually require sudden bursts of energy and quick movements. The older your grow, the more dangerous these activities become unless you have been participating regularly in appropriate physical fitness activities.

Varying Intensity, Duration, Frequency, and Mode

There is a direct relationship between the degree of cardiorespiratory improvement and the intensity, duration, and frequency of the workout sessions. These factors can be varied to reach the same results.

Age, medical limitations, excess body weight, or a combination of these may make it necessary to vary the intensity and duration components. If you can't work out at your training heart rate, then you will need more frequent workouts five to six times a week at a lower intensity and for a longer duration (45 to 60 minutes). In our program, older people and people excessively overweight start out with walking as their main exercise mode. Walking produces a lower heart rate intensity, and thus requires a longer exercise period to achieve fitness gains.

A five-day-a-week program results in greater improvements than a three-day-a-week program. However, we strongly recommend, especially for beginners, a four-day-a-week exercise schedule to lessen the chance of injury during the early stages of training. After your body adapts to regular bouts of exercise you may safely add more workouts.

Although running is a common mode of activity for cardiorespiratory improvement, some people find it boring. Even if you don't like to or may not be able to run, you can still establish a successful fitness program. You don't have to run to be fit! You can walk, swim, skip rope, or even dance (vigorously) if you wish. But the intensity, duration, and frequency of these activities must be adjusted to get beneficial results.

Remember, your goal is to achieve the results obtained by reaching a target heart rate of 75% of your heart rate reserve, for 30 minutes, four days a week. Working out at a lower heart rate requires an upward adjustment in duration, frequency, or both. Likewise, shorter exercise periods must be balanced with more workouts.

When choosing a mode, you must know how hard, how long, and how often to work out with that mode to get the desired results. The information provided in Chapters 8 through 12 will help you choose from a variety of modes. Once you have learned how you respond to various modes, you can better adjust your intensity, duration, and frequency.

The Three-Segment Workout

Most workouts for developing physical fitness consist of three essential parts: (1) the warm-up; (2) the main vigorous conditioning period; and (3) the cool-down. All three segments are necessary for a sound program.

The Warm-Up

Proper warm-up before each workout is a wise habit. In addition to preparing your body for the upcoming workout, the warm-up is a precaution against unnecessary injuries and muscle soreness. It progressively stimulates the heart and lungs, increases the blood flow, and gradually increases the temperatures of the blood and muscles. A complete warm-up will stretch the muscles and tendons in preparation for more forceful contractions. It also prepares you mentally for the strenuous workout. You should experience an overall feeling of well-being as you complete your preparation.

THE THREE SEGMENT WORKOUT

Warming Up.

The Main Conditioning Workout

Cooling Down.

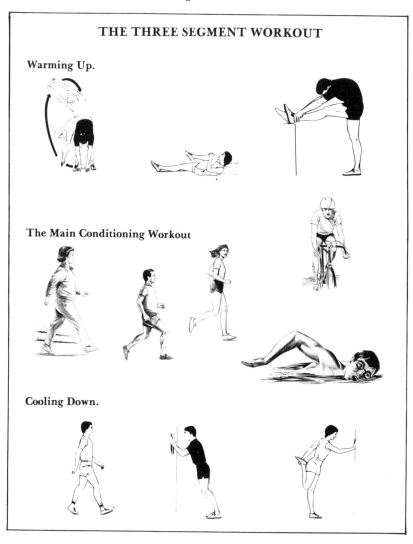

The time required for a warm-up varies with the individual. However, as soon as you begin to sweat (an indication that the temperature of the deep tissues has increased) you are probably ready for the more intense conditioning workout. Keep in mind that cool weather requires longer warm-up times.

Because of the importance of this segment of your workout, we have devoted a complete chapter to proper warming up and stretching exercises. Chapter 7 presents a sequence of 12 exercises that we have developed over the years and use daily in our program at Ball State University.

The Main Conditioning Period

After a sufficient warm-up, you are now ready for the main conditioning segment of your workout. We recommend endurance-type activities such as walking, running, bicycling, swimming, skipping rope, cross-country skiing, aerobic dancing, and other activities that are continuous and rhythmic. On some days, especially as you get in better shape, vigorous participation in your favorite sport may be used as your principal workout.

In most workouts, your exercise during this vigorous conditioning segment should be close to 75% of your heart rate reserve, as was explained earlier in this chapter. If you alternate periods of vigorous exercise with exercise of lower intensity (you will learn how to do this in later chapters), you will be able to keep from going over your target heart rate. Your peak efforts should never exceed 85 to 90% HR reserve. However, when you reach the point where your workout is without alternating periods of exercise and rest, as in continuous running or swimming, then it will be easier to judge and maintain your target heart rate without much fluctuation. It is common for those who can sustain running for 30 or more minutes to elevate their heart rate to the 85% level and be comfortable. For those on a walking program, it is unlikely you can elevate your heart rate to the 75% level. However, you can walk for a longer period to compensate.

Remember, the key is to tailor your program to your personal needs. As your fitness capacity improves over time, it will be possible to modify your workout and increase the total work accomplished in each session. *But the workout should always be set so that you feel fully recovered and rested within an hour of its completion.* At the start, your workout may last only 20 minutes, but gradually you will become accustomed to longer periods of vigorous exercise at the intensity level you have established for yourself.

The Cool-Down

The cool-down is a tapering off period after completion of the main workout. It is best accomplished by a continuation of activity at a lowered intensity level. Some highly trained individuals use intermittent running at a lower tempo as a cooling-down procedure. However, walking is a more common practice. Some of the warm-up exercises need to be repeated during cool-down.

The reason for tapering off is to allow your muscles to assist in pumping the blood from the extremities back to the heart. If you end a workout abruptly, your heart will continue to send extra blood to the muscles for a few minutes. Since the muscles are no longer contracting and helping to propel the blood back to the central circulation, blood may pool in the muscles. As a result, there may be insufficient blood for the other organs of the body. In fact, if you don't keep moving you may experience dizziness. Therefore, it is wise to keep moving to help your breathing and heart rate return to near normal before you head for a shower. Generally, a five-to-ten minute recovery period is sufficient under normal conditions. For most participants, the heart rate at the end of the cool-down should be below 100.

The Aerobics Program Vs. Ball State Fitness Program

I am often asked how our philosophy of exercise training compares with or differs from the Aerobics Program that was popularized as a formal methods of exercise over 14 years ago by Dr. Kenneth H. Cooper, then a major in the United States Air Force Medical Corp. Fundamentally, the goals of each program are to improve the endurance capacities of the heart, lungs, and muscles — to improve maximal oxygen uptake. However, they differ in that the Cooper program is based on accumulating points. When you cover a specific distance in a specific amount of time you award yourself a certain number of aerobic points based on charts devised by Dr. Cooper. He recommends a goal of 30 points per week for men and 24 points for women. In contrast, our recommendations are concerned more with exercising at a heart rate (intensity) over a period of time (duration). Such a program adapts easier to climatic conditions (e.g., heat and humidity).

Our objection to the point system is that there is too much emphasis on earning points. The method we propose is based on how your body responds to an exercise workout using your heart rate as an indicator of intensity. In other words, by monitoring your pulse rate you can structure your workouts at an effort level that is right for you. To repeat, we want you to strive to always work out well within your capabilities, but at an intensity level that adequately challenges your cardiorespiratory system. Exercising at or near a 75% HR reserve intensity provides an adequate stimulus for improving and maintaining physical fitness.

As previously mentioned, both programs are concerned with improving your aerobic capacity. Although Dr. Cooper wisely suggests in his latest book, *Aerobics Way,* that one progress "safely and slowly," he inadvertently encourages you to violate this principle when he also emphatically states, ". . . remember the objectives of aerobics is to get the required number of points per week, not to exercise in any particular way or at any particular speed or intensity."

Furthermore, periodically checking your pulse rate (rather than checking a stop watch to see if you covered a mile or more fast enough to get the points) helps you to adjust more favorably to changing conditions. Some days you may not feel up to par. On such days even though you may not be able to run, walk, or swim so fast, your pulse rate might indicate that you are adequately stressing your body. Climatic conditions such as heat and humidity will tend to make your exercise heart rate higher. The Cooper system does not readily take this into account. Therefore, using your pulse rate to monitor your exercise efforts will help keep you from overdoing it. It is a much better and safer way than striving to get a certain number of points each day.

Doctor Cooper's claim that if you achieve 30 points a week, no matter how you do it, you are physically fit, can be questioned. It was briefly mentioned at the outset of this chapter that our suggestions for training are in line with the recommended guidelines published by the American College of Sports Medicine. Based on this position paper (90 scientifically documented experiments), 30 aerobic points a week is a minimal effort, if that.

The point system has also been open to criticism because of apparent discrepancies when points are assessed for a wide variety of activities. Despite what Dr. Cooper claims, there is not sufficient scientific data to support his system. For example, there is no published evidence to my knowledge that playing volleyball for an hour can be equated to running a mile in between eight and ten minutes.

Doctor Cooper based his tables of aerobic points on energy costs. Mistakenly, Dr. Cooper implies that if you run a mile faster, you will burn more energy for that mile. It is true that the rate of energy expenditure per minute is higher as you run faster. However, the total energy required to cover a mile is quite similar whether you run it at twelve minutes or eight minutes. Although Dr. Cooper recognizes that "there are simply too many variables involved to establish an exact calories-per-aerobic-point-figure," he does suggest that you won't go too far wrong by estimating a calorie expenditure of 20 calories per aerobic point (600 calories for a 30-point week). By contrast, in our program the eventual goal of 30 minutes of continuous exercise at 75% heart rate reserve intensity for a minimum of four days is equal to as few as 50 to almost 100 of Dr. Cooper points, depending upon your level of fitness. In fact, many of our people easily accumulate over 100 points or 2,000 calories a week. Let me emphasize: *you need more than 600 calories (30 points) a week of exercise.* In fact, as you begin to get in shape so that you can sustain a 75% HR intensity for 20 to 30 minutes, you will eventually be able to burn between 300 and 400 calories per session. Thus, a minimum for our program is 1,200 calories per week (4 × 300 calories) or 60 aerobic points, if you wish. However, as you keep going, you will most likely be capable of burning close to 500 calories per workout, or 2,000 or more calories per week (100 plus aerobic points). And, you do not have to race against a clock to achieve your goals.

Summary

In summary, working at your 75% HR reserve is mostly aerobic, so don't worry about how fast you go (whether you swim, run, or cycle). Your heart's response to your workout should be your main concern. To most people who do not exercise, the recommendations in this chapter may seem unreasonable and impossible. Let me assure you, *you can do it!* Whether you want to walk, run, cycle, or swim, the programs outlined in this book can help you. But you must be willing to devote the necessary time and effort to your fitness training if you want to reap the benefits.

Today, nearly everyone preaches the virtues of physical fitness, yet many of these same people do not themselves maintain a regular fitness program. Two primary reasons for this failure to maintain individual fitness are not knowing: (1) how much exercise is enough, and (2) the kinds of exercise that work best for physical fitness. In fact, many writers on physical fitness have neglected to take a firm stand on recommending physical fitness activities. One frequently hears vague statements, such as, "There are many ways to develop fitness," "Do your own thing," "Choose whatever activity you enjoy," or "Don't overdo it," "Don't sweat." Such suggestions are chaotic and groundless and confuse the reader. Of course there are different ways to develop cardiorespiratory fitness. Nevertheless, you must exert yourself, in a continuous and rhythmic activity at a substantial level of exertion for at least 30 minutes. And you must adhere to this program regularly.

The key is the heart rate. It must be pushed high enough and held there long enough for cardiorespiratory conditioning to take place. Let's be clear about it: it takes effort to be physically fit. This does not mean punishing, exhaustive exercise, but rather a workout that is well within your present physical capacity (75% HR reserve).

The exercise charts in the chapters that follow have been developed from our knowledge and actual experience of what it takes for people to become fit, regardless of their present physical status. Our charts represent carefully planned steps to guide you through the early stages of getting in shape, and most important, at an intensity that is right for you. Eventually you will reach the point where you will not need the charts. At that point you will be ready to assume the responsibility of continuing your own workouts and maintaining your new status of being fit.

Before beginning an exercise program, it's essential to know your physical capacity or fitness level. The next chapter assists you in appraising your current level of fitness and directs you to activities that are best for your given abilities.

chapter five

Determining Your Level of Fitness

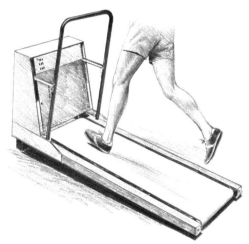

How healthy are you? How do you know whether you are in shape? What is your current level of fitness? Is it safe for you to exercise? Before beginning a program of exercise, you should find the answers to these questions.

Taking a battery of physical fitness tests will provide answers to such questions. The results of the tests will help you set personal fitness goals. When you repeat the tests after a few months of training, you can check the effectiveness of your exercise training. Test results provide an effective incentive for getting and staying in shape.

If you are in doubt about your state of health, first check with a medical doctor (your personal physician, if you have one) before engaging in any testing or exercise training. If you can find a doctor who regularly engages in exercise training (running, swimming, cycling), you are more apt to get understanding help and encouragement.

Exercise Tolerance Test

Is it important to take an exercise tolerance test before starting a fitness program? Most health professionals say yes. However, many people avoid such testing. It is probably not practical for everyone who desires to exercise to get such a comprehensive physical evaluation. However, if you can take an exercise tolerance test, we urge you to do so.

The need for a physical evaluation becomes more evident when such factors as age, current health status, family history, and present exercise habits are considered. For example, do you huff and puff while climbing stairs? Are you fatigued after mowing the lawn or doing routine household chores? Do you, at times, experience chest pains during exertion? If so, you are badly out of shape.

If you have not been active in recent years, it is wise to have a physical examination before undergoing any type of fitness training.

The next table provides a quick estimate of your need to take a physical examination. Important factors are listed, and beside each is a row of choices from which you can pick the one most applicable to you. For example, if you are 45, you would circle the number 3 in the age row. After carefully circling the appropriate box in each row, total the numbers circled. This sum of scores represents an approximation of your present health. The higher the score, the higher the risk of exercising and the greater the need to see a doctor. (See page 66 for scoring instructions.)

HEALTH STATUS INVENTORY TABLE

Age	10 to 20	21 to 30	31 to 40	41 to 50	51 and above
	0	0	1	3	5
Genetics	No known history of heart disease in family	One relative with heart disease over 50	Two relatives with heart disease over 50	One relative under 50 with heart disease	Two relatives under 50 with heart disease
	0	1	2	4	5
Fatness[1]	Male 13% or below / Female 20% or below	14-16% / 21-23%	17-20% / 24-26%	21-24% / 27-29%	25% and above / 30% and above
	0	1	2	3	4
Smoking	Non-smoker	Cigar and/or pipe	10 cigarettes or less a day	20 cigarettes or less a day	more than 20 cigarettes a day
	0	1	3	5	7
Blood[2] Pressure	Systolic 120 or lower	Systolic 130-120	Systolic 140-130	Systolic 150-140	Systolic 150 or above
	0	1	2	3	5
Exercise	Regularly run, cycle, swim 30 min. three times a week	Heavy physical work; some sports playing	Light physical work or limited physical exercise	Sedentary work; light recreational activity	Sedentary work, sitting most of day; little walking
	0	1	3	4	5
Sex	Female under 40	Male under 40	Female over 40	Male over 40	Over 50
	0	1	2	3	5

On pages 86-95, instructions for estimating your fatness are provided.
Hopefully you have had your blood pressure checked recently; if not, we highly recommend that you do!

If You Score

0 to 6	It is most likely safe to participate. You may want to go through some of the self-tests to assess your present physical status.
7 to 15	It is probably safe for you to begin one of the starter programs; you should check with your physician first before undergoing the self-testing battery.
16 to 25	You should see a physician about taking an exercise tolerance test. During the early stages of training it would be best to begin with a walking program.
26 and up	You need to see a physician. You should take an exercise tolerance test. If a tolerance test is not feasible, begin the walking program in Chapter 8, but only with the advice of your physician. Use the walk test for an indication of where to begin.

The table below provides a series of questions as another means to help you detect any hidden health problem or any impending risks of exercise.

MEDICAL SCREENING QUESTIONNAIRE

Answer yes or no to each question.

_____ **1.** Do you ever experience sensations of pain, pressure, or tightness in the center of your chest under the breastbone?

_____ **2.** Do you ever experience a pain in the throat region or running down the left arm?

_____ **3.** Do you ever get dizzy, lightheaded, or even faint during light to moderate exercise?

		MEDICAL SCREENING QUESTIONNAIRE (cont'd)

_____ **4.** Have you ever felt an abnormal heart action such as irregular beats, a fluttering, or a jumping in the chest or neck?

_____ **5.** Do you have diabetes? High blood sugar?

_____ **6.** Are you taking medication to control blood pressure?

_____ **7.** Do you have above normal levels of fats in your blood (cholesterol, triglycerides, low density lipoproteins)?

_____ **8.** Do you smoke more than 10 cigarettes daily?

_____ **9.** Do you have any known orthopedic (bone, joint, muscular) problems that could be further harmed by exercise?

_____ **10.** Are you 30 to 40 pounds overweight? (Clue: How much heavier are you than your high school weight, assuming you had no weight problems then?)

_____ **11.** Do you easily get out of breath and have to stop your activities while others easily carry on?

If you answer no to all the questions, the likelihood of your having any hidden health problems is very slight. If you answer yes to any of the questions, consulting with a physician would be in your best interest before beginning your personal fitness training, especially for those over 40 and recently inactive.

Who Do You Go to for a Good Evaluation?

The basis for exercise tolerance testing and exercise prescription has been well established by the American Heart Association and the American College of Sports Medicine. Unfortunately, most physicians lack the appropriate background and equipment to conduct exercise testing. Having an M.D. degree does not necessarily assure competency to supervise exercise tolerance testing or to provide an exercise prescription. Exercise physiology and training in conducting functional exercise tests have not been part of most physician's medical education. Traditionally, medical education has emphasized the treating of acute illness. Consequently the average physician has little interest or time to work out detailed exercise prescriptions. Fortunately, medical curriculums are now dealing with these skills, and more and more physicians are becoming knowledgeable about physical fitness and the benefits of regular exercise.

In recent years, with the increased interest in physical fitness, more centers are being developed that have the capability and staff for administering fitness evaluations. Workshops and college curriculums aimed at training exercise specialists are now more frequent. More physical educators, health educators, and physicians are being trained in the basic knowledge and skills for administering fitness evaluations and conducting effective exercise programs.

If your physician is unable to administer an exercise tolerance test, he or she will tell you whether you need such a test and may even refer you to a reputable exercise testing center. Many universities, YMCAs, community centers, and private fitness centers are now providing quality testing programs. In most cases, these centers employ medical doctors, exercise specialists, and technicians who have achieved competency for such work. Many of these professionals have met the rigorous American College of Sports Medicine certification standards.

I am a member of the Preventive-Rehabilitative Exercise Committee of the American College of Sports Medicine. This committee has been responsible for setting certification qualifications and standards. As of the fall, 1981, 126 program directors, 243 exercise specialists, and 983 exercise technologists have passed extensive written and practical exams indicating a high level of competence for working in preventive and rehabilitative exercise programs.

What To Expect From an Evaluation

One of the purposes of an evaluation is to provide information that will help you design a personalized program of exercise. Such information can be determined by having your body's response to exercise checked.

An evaluation for exercise clearance generally follows a standard format. First, your family history is reviewed along with an up-to-date medical history. Information such as cigarette smoking, alcohol consumption, and your physical activity habits are noted and recorded. A standard electrocardiogram (ECG) is recorded and interpreted to detect any abnormalities. For most people a resting ECG is not likely to disclose heart disease. However, graded exercise testing may reveal the possibility of disease of the arteries of the heart. Blood pressure and heart rate are measured while sitting. In many instances, blood samples are drawn and analyzed to determine the amount of fats (cholesterol, triglycerides, lipoproteins) and sugar (glucose) in your blood. Your weight, height, and often the percentage of your body fat is measured. Although all this information is not used directly for planning your exercise workouts, such information provides much insight into your overall health and alerts you to any impairment that may limit your exercise training.

The next table lists the basics of three standard testing formats. Plan A is the most thorough and preferred format for testing physical fitness and risk factors for coronary heart disease. In contrast, Plan C provides minimal information and can be self-administered. Later in this chapter we will show how to test yourself to gain this information.

The exercise tolerance test (often referred to as a graded exercise test) is designed to determine the functional capacity of your body (how it responds to exercise) and is generally conducted on a treadmill or a bicycle ergometer. The treadmill, although initially more expensive to purchase for the testing center, has the advantage of using a familiar mode of exercise — walking or running. The bicycle ergometer (a stationary exercise bike) is relatively less expensive, but most people are not accustomed to riding a bike. Pedaling a bike often results in fatigue of the thigh muscles at relatively low exercise rates. Walking and running on the treadmill bring into play large muscle masses resulting in less localized fatigue of the legs during testing.

Many standardized tolerance test formats have been developed for the treadmill and bicycle ergometer. Each test will begin with the subject exercising at a low level of exertion, gradually and systematically increasing effort over time to some defined end-point. The increased effort is achieved by either increasing the speed or incline (or both) of the treadmill or increasing the pedal resistance of the bike. In some labs the test may be completed at some predetermined submaximal level of exertion and the results used to predict maximal performance. In our laboratory we prefer using the treadmill. Our test continues until the subject indicates that maximal level has been reached; that is, the subject can go no longer. Through preliminary tests (such as medical and

Testing Formats

	PLAN A	PLAN B	PLAN C
Cardiorespiratory			
Rest	ECG	ECG	
	Sitting heart rate	Sitting HR	Sitting HR
	Blood pressure	Blood pressure	
Exercise	Functional exer- cise tolerance test to max.	Functional exer- cise tolerance test, submaximal (predicts max.)	Walking or walk-run field test
	Blood pressure	Blood pressure	
	ECG monitoring	ECG monitoring	
Body fat analysis			
	Height	Height	Height
	Weight	Weight	Weight
	Skinfold measures	Skinfold measures	Estimate of
	Estimate of % fat	Estimate of % fat	% fat
	Determine goals and desired weights	Determine goals and desired weights	Determine goals and desired weights
Blood measures			
	Cholesterol	Cholesterol	
	Triglycerides	Triglycerides	
	Lipoproteins		
	Glucose		
Muscular strength (optional) **and endurance**			
	Bent-leg sit-ups (one minute)	Bent-leg sit-ups (one minute)	Bent-leg sit-ups (one minute)
	Push-ups	Push-ups	Push-ups
Flexibility (optional)			
	Sit and reach test	Sit and reach test	Sit and reach test

activity history, blood pressure, fat percentage) a physiological capability is estimated that allows us to set a format that will safely fulfill the intended purpose of the test.

For older people who have been inactive, we commonly start them walking at a pace of about three miles per hour (for some even slower). The choice of speed depends on the estimated capabilities; for example, a woman with short legs would most likely walk at the slower speed. Generally, this starting speed for walking is low enough so that most people go through several stages of progressively increased workloads which may include running before the voluntary end-point is reached. After a few minutes of level exercise (essentially a warm-up), the grade or incline of the treadmill is adjusted upward 2% every two minutes. This sequence continues, increasing the amount of effort required at each grade, until the subject can't supply the energy required to meet the muscular demand—the person's tolerance for exercise has been achieved. At this time, the maximal heart rate has been reached. For the normal, healthy person, the end-point will be fatigue, most likely a combination of breathlessness and tired leg muscles.

Throughout the testing process the exercise electrocardiogram is being monitored on an oscilloscope (an instrument with a TV-type screen that displays the electrical output of one's heart) and tracings are recorded during each minute of exercise and recovery. During the tolerance test a medical doctor is present to watch for any evidence of impaired heart function. Generally, for persons 35 years of age or older a physician should be present, especially for people who have been previously inactive and have blood pressure, weight, or other problems that suggest possible risks to exercise. The test will usually be discontinued before the subject reaches the physiological maximal performance if he or she shows any serious abnormal responses such as chest discomfort, faintness, or an abnormal electrocardiogram.

Another appropriate function that is monitored, especially during a walking test, is blood pressure. The measurement of blood pressure during exercise is difficult because of the presences of extraneous sounds. However, with the older, inactive person, the monitoring of blood pressure will alert the testing team to how the heart muscle is adapting to the increased workload. In short, a falling systolic pressure with increased workloads suggests some failure of the heart to adapt and necessitates discontinuing the test.

At Ball State University (and at some other research labs) one additional dimension is added to the testing. Throughout the test the sub-

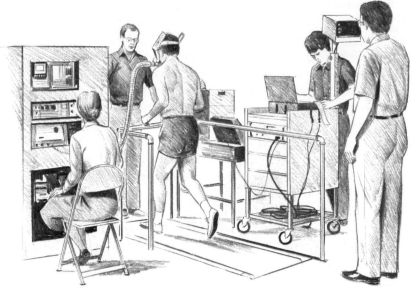

Figure 10. Exercise tolerance testing in the lab.

ject is hooked up to our respiratory analysis system, as shown. This involves breathing room air through a mouthpiece with a nose clip attached so that all exhaled air can be collected. The volume of air breathed in is measured, and samples of expired air are collected and the oxygen and carbon dioxide content measured. These measurements are used to calculate the amount of oxygen used during each stage of the test and to determine the maximal amount of oxygen used. Maximal oxygen uptake can be expressed as maximal MET capacity. One MET represents the rate of energy at rest. Therefore, maximal METs represents your highest energy capacity in multiples above rest. For example, a 10 MET capacity means an energy capacity of ten times the capacity when sitting in a chair. Later in this book, you will learn the importance of knowing your maximal MET capacity. The measurement of maximal oxygen uptake is the best indicator of the fitness and functional capacity of the heart and lungs. (Refer to Chapter 2 for a physiological explanation of maximal oxygen uptake.) This additional equipment is cumbersome and distracting but produces valuable results.

Is the Exercise Tolerance Test Safe?

The exercise tolerance test, such as the one just described, is quite safe, if properly conducted. The heart's activity is monitored by an electrocardiograph along with blood pressure measurements. Any irregularities of the heart's response to exercise becomes evident immediately when properly monitored.

The exercise tolerance test on either a treadmill or bike is frightening at first. Let's not kid ourselves, going to our "max" is taxing. Realizing that we do not have to exercise at max each day to get in shape helps us get through this ordeal. Remember, the purpose of this test is to determine your maximal capacity so that you can set your exercise workouts at a comfortable but stimulating level (usually 75% of your maximum capability) to ensure beneficial changes. Although the testing procedure may be somewhat uncomfortable, it is safe, and the resulting data provides in-depth insight into your current level of fitness.

Detecting Heart Disease

There is some controversy today in the medical profession regarding reliability of an exercise tolerance test for detecting coronary heart disease. Recent medical data suggest that the electrocardiographic (ECG) response to the exercise tolerance test is a poor predictor of coronary disease in a healthy population. The key phrase of the previous statement is "healthy population." We can agree somewhat with this since our main purpose is to determine a person's fitness capabilities so we can assist them in developing a reasonable program of exercise training. However, during a testing session we might observe abnormal rhythms or changes in someone's ECG. The degree of these abnormalities, the intensity of exercise that provokes them, and a lowering of blood pressure due to increasing workloads are strong indicators of the likelihood of coronary heart disease. Our experiences in taking people to their subjective maximums have at times detected such signs of possible heart disease. We inform them that this is not cause for alarm, but it is reason for concern. After careful assessment of each individual case, we may suggest further medical tests to determine in more detail the significance of this information. Each case must be dealt with separately. Often, further diagnostic testing has revealed blocked arteries in the heart. Some of these cases have required open-heart surgery and many of these people are now exercising (walking and running) regularly.

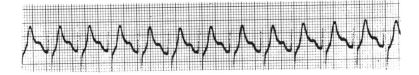

Fortunately, many of these people have been encouraged by their cardiologists to return to our program. We make adjustments in their workouts accordingly, and in most cases, they progress favorably through the stages of our training program.

After people have been informed of an impaired heart function many are motivated to alter their lifestyles. In other words, smokers cease smoking, fat people modify their eating habits, and the inactive take up endurance-type exercise.

Interpreting Test Results

If you take an exercise tolerance test, you need to know how to interpret the results in order to get the most out of the information gained. Most centers will provide all the necessary information in a personal profile. If they don't, *request it!* You need this information in order to more effectively utilize the endurance-type programs presented in the following chapters.

The profile sheet shown in the next table lists the basic information needed. With these data you can easily determine your fitness level and your target or training heart rate.

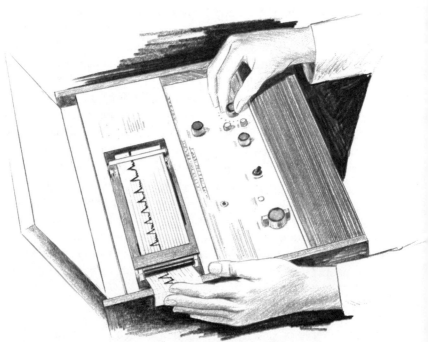

PHYSICAL FITNESS PROFILE

MUSTS   **Sitting Heart Rate**   _____ beats/minute

           Maximal Heart Rate   _____ beats/minute

           Maximal Oxygen Uptake[1]   _____ml/kg•minute

           Maximal MET Level   _____METS[2]

HELPFUL   *(But not necessary for designing a plan of exercise*
           training)

           Body Weight   _____ lbs   (_____kg)

           Skinfolds[3]: _____

           % Body fat[4]: _____

           Sitting Blood Pressure   _____mmHg

           Cholesterol   _____mg%

           Triglycerides   _____mg%

           High Density Lipoprotein   _____mg%

           Glucose (Blood Sugar)   _____mg%

---

[1]Many labs are not equipped to measure this, but tables are available to assist the lab specialists in estimating your maximal capacity. Be sure to request this information.

[2]One MET = 3.5 ml/kg•min, the rate of energy at rest.

[3]See Appendix A for using skinfold calipers (if you have access to them).

[4]If you cannot have your percentage of fat determined in a laboratory situation, a simple method for estimating it is provided on page 87.

Turn to the table on pages 78 and 79, locate your MET value, and note your recommended starting point in the various charts. This information is needed in order to use effectively the exercise training charts in later chapters.

Is It Safe To Proceed Without a Tolerance Test?

If it is not feasible for you to get a comprehensive physical examination with a functional exercise tolerance test, then the next best thing is to have your family doctor check you and then to conduct a self-test with some of the tests that are explained in the next section of this chapter.

The approval of your physician and the knowledge that you have no health problems can bolster your confidence to proceed into some self-

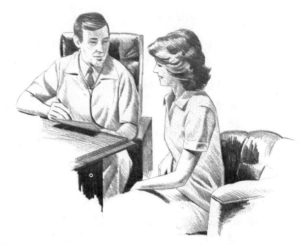

testing. However, from a practical viewpoint, there are not enough physicians or qualified exercise specialists to examine all the people who wish to begin vigorous exercise training. Certainly not all the many thousands of people who make up the running boom were subjected to an exercise tolerance test or had the approval of a doctor before beginning their training program. So even though it's preferable to have a physician's consent, it may not be practical. If you answered no to all of the questions in the medical screening questionnaire, then it's probably safe for you to proceed with the self-tests.

Doctor P.O. Astrand, a world-renowned exercise physiologist and director of the Institute of Work Physiology in Stockholm, says this about medical examinations: "The question is frequently raised whether a medical examination is advisable before commencing a training program. Certainly, anyone doubtful about his (or her) state of health should consult a physician . . . (however) in principle there is less risk in activity than continuous inactivity, and . . . it is more advisable to pass a careful medical examination if one intends to be sedentary (inactive) in order to establish whether one's state of health is good enough to stand the inactivity." Enough said?

Self-Testing

The self-test battery consists of a group of tests to measure your cardiorespiratory endurance, estimate the fat content of your body, and measure your strength, muscular endurance, and flexibility. Directions follow for a walking or a run-walk test to enable you to select a suitable and safe starting point for your cardiorespiratory endurance training (whether it will be walking, running, cycling, or swimming). Once you have completed this test or tests, you need only refer to the table on pages 78, 79 to determine the proper place (based on your estimated maximal METS) for you to begin your rhythmic endurance-type exercise training. Knowing your fitness capabilities (maximal METS) will help you use the exercise charts effectively. These tests will give you at least some idea of what kind of shape you are in before you start.

Cardiorespiratory Endurance Tests

Walking test. If you are over 35, you should first do the walking test. This is especially wise if you are considerably overweight, and have been inactive in recent months.

To test yourself, you need a timing device; a stopwatch or wrist watch with a second hand is satisfactory. You also need to find an area where the distance is known. A measured track at your local high school or YW/YMCA is a possibility, or you may want to measure the distance on a street in your neighborhood; use your car odometer to measure the distance for 1 mile, 1½ miles, 2 miles, and 3 miles.

If you are going to test yourself outdoors, choose a day that is clear and not below freezing or above 80°. In some areas it may be necessary to walk in the early morning to avoid the heat and humidity. Proceed to your previously selected route. As you begin walking, start the stopwatch or note the time on your watch (it's easier if you start with the second hand on 12). Walk as briskly as you can. If you begin to tire early, slow up. If you cannot complete the mile or if you cannot complete it in under 25 minutes, then the test is completed. If you reach the

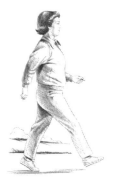

DETERMINING YOUR FITNESS LEVEL

Fitness Level in Maximal METS$_1$		Recommended Starting Points For		
		Walking or Running	Swimming	Cycling$_2$
If you can walk 1.0 mile:				
in longer than 25 min.	4 or below	Walking Program Chart 1, Step 1	Swim Chart 1, Step 1	Cycle at a comfortable pace for 12 min.
in less than 25 min. but longer than 20 min.	4.5	Walking Program Chart 1, Step 3		THEN:
If you can walk 1.5 mile:				Increase by 4 min. every two workouts until you can cover 30 to 40 min. with ease; then begin at Cycling Chart 1, Step 1
in less than 30 min. but longer than 26 min.	5	Walking Program Chart 1, Step 5	Swim Chart 1, Step 3	
in less than 26 min. but longer than 23 min.	5.5	Walking Program Chart 1, Step 7		
If you can walk 2.0 miles:				
in less than 40 min. but longer than 35 min.	6	Walking Program Chart 2, Step 9	Swim Chart 1, Step 5	
in less than 35 min. but longer than 30 min.	6.5	Walking Program Chart 2, Step 13		

DETERMINING YOUR FITNESS LEVEL (cont'd)

	METS	Program	Swim	Cycling
If you can walk 3.0 miles: in less than 52:30 min. but longer than 45 min.	7	Walking Program Chart 3A or 3B, Step 17	Swim Chart 2, Step 1	Cycling Chart 1, Step 1
in less than 45 min.	7.5	Walking Program Chart 3A or 3B, Step 19	Swim Chart 2, Step 3	Cycling Chart 1, Step 3
If you can run-walk 2.0 miles: in longer than 25 min.	8	Run-Walk Program Chart 1, Step 1	Swim Chart 2, Step 5	Cycling Chart 1, Step 5
in less than 24:59 min. but longer than 23 min.	8.5	Run-Walk Program Chart 1, Step 6	Swim Chart 3, Step 1	Cycling Chart 1, Step 7
in less than 22:59 min. but longer than 21 min.	9	Run-Walk Program Chart 2, Step 1	Swim Chart 3, Step 3	Cycling Chart 1, Step 9
in less than 20:59 min. but longer than 19 min.	9.5	Run-Walk Program Chart 2, Step 6	Swim Chart 3, Step 5	Cycling Chart 2, Step 1

[1] Maximal METS represents your Functional Fitness Level; if you were able to undergo an exercise tolerance test, be sure you find out your Maximal MET value whether it was estimated or actually measured.

[2] If your Maximal MET level is below 7, first become accustomed to cycling for a sustained period before using the charts. See instructions above and in Chapter 11.

mile in less than 20 minutes, keep going for another half mile. If you reach the 1½ mile point in less than 30 minutes, keep walking. Your goal is now two miles in less than 40 minutes. If you reach this goal, then keep going and try to reach three miles in 60 minutes.

If you can cover three miles in 60 minutes or less, you have two options. First you can check the fitness level table on pages 78, 79 and determine your starting point; second, on another day, you can try to run-walk a distance of two miles. This second effort may give you a more accurate idea of your capability and allow you to start at a higher level on the charts. Instead of walking, alternate running and walking for two miles, noting the time you take to complete the distance. I should emphasize that this test is not meant to be "all-out." Avoid reaching the stage of feeling breathless. In fact, we want you to keep the intensity below 75% of your heart rate reserve. After completing the two-mile run-walk, note your time, and check the fitness table to determine your estimated fitness level and starting points for the various exercise modes. Keep in mind that this table has been designed to assist those of you who have been very inactive and to help you determine a safe and reasonable starting point.

For those who are young or who have been quite active recently, the running tests that follow may be a more appropriate means of determining your fitness level.

The Running Tests

The amount of time it takes you to cover a distance of 1½ to 2 miles is an acceptable measure for approximating your maximal MET value (aerobic capacity) and fitness level. A person who is in better physical condition should be able to cover the distance in a faster time than a person in poor condition. A minimum distance of 1½ miles or a time period of 12 to 15 minutes of continuous effort has been established as the minimum for adequately estimating your aerobic capacity. However, covering the distance by running should not be done by the inactive and untrained person. Running the distance is the best and easiest way to gain information about your fitness level if you have been regularly exercising and haven't taken an exercise tolerance test. Again, you should not engage in this test if you have been deskbound and inactive in recent years. The 1½- or 2-mile tests are primarily for people who are accustomed to running the distances on a regular basis.

After you have been training and have completed the walking and run-walk charts, you may wish to test yourself using the running tests to see how you score. These tests can give you some idea on how you are progressing.

For younger people and those who can run comfortably for 15 to 20 minutes continuously, being able to run 1½ to 2 miles *all out* can give you some excellent feedback on your cardiorespiratory fitness. Since there are variations in aerobic capacities between men and women, two running tests are presented here. The 1½-mile test is for women and the 2-mile test is for men.

For men, running two miles in 10 or 12 minutes is a super rating, 12 to 14 minutes is excellent, and 14 to 16 minutes is good. For women, running 1.5 miles faster than 11.5 minutes is super, 11.5 to 13 minutes is excellent, and 13 to 14.5 minutes is good.

The times to run the 1½-mile distance all out for women and the 2-miles distance for men correlate well with actual values of maximal oxygen uptake determined on the treadmill. Therefore, estimates of your aerobic capacity are given in accordance with your running times (see the tables on pages 82, 83). Although these data (compiled in our lab) are based on young adults, these values tend to hold true for older people as well. This is especially true for people who use running as their training mode.

One word of caution, do not attempt any all out runs until you have become accustomed to running such distances on a regular basis.

Evaluating Your Body Fat and Body Shape

Many people desire to establish good nutritional and exercise habits for enhancing the natural proportions of their body. In fact, wanting to *look* good is a major motivation for most people who exercise and watch their weight. We all want to be admired and attractive to others, whether we wish to admit it or not. Our experiences at Ball State clearly show that the principal reason people begin an exercise program is discontent with the shape of their bodies.

A person's sex, age, and genetic background can account for individual variations in muscular build and the distribution of fat deposits on the body. Men and women do not put on fat (or lose it) in the same places. Some people were destined to be chunky, but they don't have to be fat. Fatness runs in families, but we don't know how much this

2-MILE RUNNING TEST FOR MEN

FITNESS CATEGORY	2.0 MILE TIME	ESTIMATED MAXIMAL OXYGEN UPTAKE EQUIVALENTS	APPROXIMATE MAXIMAL METS
Super	Faster than 12:00	55 ml/kg•min or higher	15.7 Plus
Excellent	12:00 to 13:59	54.9 to 50 ml/kg•min	15.6 to 14.3
Excellent to Good	14:00 to 15:59	49.9 to 45 ml/kg•min	14.2 to 12.9
Good to Fair	16:00 to 17:59	44.9 to 40 ml/kg•min	12.8 to 11.4
Fair to Poor	18:00 to 19:59	39.9 to 35 ml/kg•min	11.3 to 10.0
Poor	20:00 or slower	34.9 or lower	9.9 or lower

1.5-MILE RUNNING TEST FOR WOMEN

FITNESS CATEGORY	1.5 MILE TIME	ESTIMATED MAXIMAL OXYGEN UPTAKE EQUIVALENTS	APPROXIMATE MAXIMAL METS
Super	Faster than 11:30	52.5 ml/kg•min or higher	15 Plus
Excellent	11:30 to 12:59	52.4 to 47.5 ml/kg•min	14.9 to 13.6
Excellent to Good	13:00 to 14:29	46.4 to 42.5 ml/kg•min	13.5 to 12.1
Good to Fair	14:30 to 15:59	42.4 to 37.5 ml/kg•min	12.0 to 10.7
Fair to Poor	16:00 to 17:59	37.4 to 32.5 ml/kg•min	10.6 to 9.3
Poor	18:00 or slower	31.4 or lower	9.2 or lower

tendency to be fat is inherited or results from eating habits formed in the home. However, it is known that as we age we tend to lose muscle tissue, and often put on excess fat. Exercise can be an important means for controlling your body fat and overall body build. Furthermore, a well-balanced body shape reflects self-confidence and pride. Exercise can develop your muscles into pleasing shapes and contours. In addition, exercise can redistribute your weight by toning up muscles (making them firmer) and by aiding you in losing excess fat. Let's see how you measure up!

How fat are you? Being overweight because of a preponderance of bone and muscle does not have the same meaning as being overweight because of excess fat tissue. In terms of the popular standard height-weight tables used by insurance companies, over-weight does not necessarily mean excess fatness. Fatness refers to the body's fat stores. How fat you are depends on both the size and the number of your fat cells.

Body fat and lean body weight can be measured quite accurately in the laboratory. There is an underwater weighing technique based on the principle that a person with more muscle tissue and less body fat will weigh more in water. Fat floats, giving the body more buoyancy. A higher body density means a lower percentage of fat.

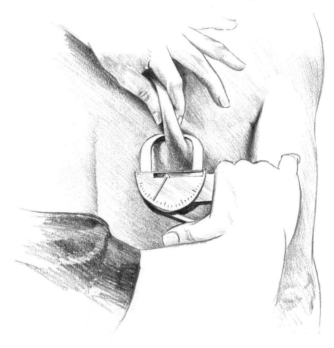

Because of the elaborate equipment, complex procedures, and substantial time required to test each individual, under water weighing methods are not widely used. As a result, researchers have developed other means for estimating body fat that are closely related to the complex laboratory techniques. Fortunately, a simple method using skinfold calipers is suitable for determining the percentage of lean tissue and fat in the body.

Many researchers have developed formulas for estimating body density using skinfold and in some cases girth measurements as predictors. If you have the opportunity to be measured at a fitness center or in a doctor's office, these measurements will be helpful in providing a good estimate of your relative body fat (percentage of fat). If you have access to skinfold calipers (some inexpensive ones available for under $10 are adequate), refer to Appendix A for instructions on measuring and computing your fat percent.

For most people the opportunity to be measured for body fat in a laboratory setting is limited. Even if you have access to skinfold calipers, unless the person measuring you has considerable experience in accurately using calipers, your values may not be very accurate. As an alternative, we have devised tables based on your height and a simple estimate of your degree of muscularity to estimate not only your ideal weight but also your percent of body fat. The ideal weight tables on pages 88, 89 are based on men and women in our Ball State Fitness Program who have been very active and who have trim bodies. The tables represent weights for various heights with what we consider to be desired percentages of fat, namely, 12% for men and 18% for women.

sider the quality of your body weight. A physically fit individual tends to have firmer muscles. The popular height-weight tables disregard your body composition. Therefore, you may weigh more than the charts indicate, but not necessarily have excess fat on your body. This is not to imply that our tables are 100% accurate, but we have tested them with other methods and they provide a reasonable estimate of fatness. The trick, of course, is to determine your degree of muscularity.

Another factor that can affect these estimates is the weight of your skeleton or bones. It is well established that men generally have heavier bones, more muscle mass and, less stored fat (fat under the skin and around organs for protection) than women. Women possess more essential fat (fat stored in the bones, organs, and the breast tissue) than men. Therefore, a trim woman will have a higher fat percentage than a trim man. Based on our experiences with thousands of measurements, we have found the body fat percentage of 12% for men and 18% for women represent a desired trimness. This is true whether you are genetically chunky or skinny.

In order to estimate your muscularity, all you need to do is measure the girth of your calf muscle at its widest circumference. With this measurement (in inches), refer to the table on page 88 to see if you have low, medium, or high muscularity.

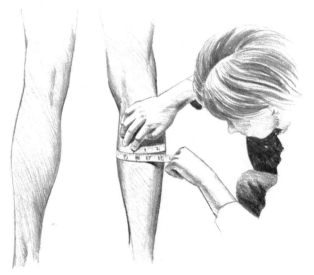

Now refer to the ideal weight tables and find your barefoot height in inches in the table and move across to the column for your degree of muscularity.

The weight in that column is an estimate of your ideal weight. You must realize that this is an estimate and weighing a few pounds above or below your value isn't worth quibbling over. We must point out that these tables lose some of their accuracy for those who are quite tall or quite short. Nevertheless, they provide a reasonable goal for a desired body weight.

You may have doubts about using the girth of your calf muscle as a means to classify your body type. If you wish, try an alternative method by determining your bone structure. Simply measure your wrist at its smallest circumference with a tape measure. Refer to the table on page 89 to see if you have low, medium, or large bone structure. Just as you did with the girth measurement, refer to the ideal weight tables and use the column corresponding to low, medium, and large across from your barefoot height.

Once you have determined your ideal weight from the tables and your present weight on a scale, you can use the following simple formula to estimate your percentage of body fat.

For Women:
$$\frac{\text{Existing Weight} - (.82 \times \text{Ideal Weight})}{\text{Existing Weight}} \times 100 = \% \text{ Fat}$$

For Men:
$$\frac{\text{Existing Weight} - (.88 \times \text{Ideal Weight})}{\text{Existing Weight}} \times 100 = \% \text{ Fat}$$

Here is an example of how the formula works. A man who is 70 inches tall and weighs 185 pounds classifies himself as medium muscularity. Referring to the ideal weight table we find that an ideal weight for a 70-inch, medium-muscular man is 165 pounds. Along with this value (165 pounds) and his existing weight (185 pounds), we can easily figure his percent fat.

$$\frac{185 - (.88 \times 165)}{185} = \frac{185 - (145.2)}{185} = \frac{39.8}{185} = .215$$

$.215 \times 100 = 21.5\% \text{ Fat}$

You might ask, "What if my ideal weight is higher than my existing weight?" This is quite possible if you are in good shape. Many runners, cyclists, and other athletes will tend to be lower than the 18% or 12% values we recommend. To clarify this, let's take a 64-inch, 110-pound woman of medium muscularity. Referring to the ideal weight table we note that an ideal weight for her is 116 pounds. With this information we can now calculate her percent formula:

$$\frac{110 - (.82 \times 116)}{110} = \frac{110 - (95.1)}{110} = \frac{14.9}{110} = .135$$

$.135 \times 100 = 13.5\% \text{ Fat}$

The resulting value of 13.5% is quite possible for a well-trained woman.

As stated earlier, laboratory methods for determining body fat percentages are not readily available. We strongly feel that our methods for predicting a desired weight and percentage of body fat is a

CALF GIRTH MEASUREMENTS		
DEGREE OF MUSCULARITY (estimate)	WOMEN (inches)	MEN (inches)
Low	12½ and below	14 and below
Medium	12½–13½	14–15½
High	13½ and up	15½ and up

IDEAL WEIGHTS FOR MEN
Based on 12% Body Fat
and Degree of Muscularity

HEIGHT (inches)	DEGREE OF MUSCULARITY		
	Low	Medium	High
60	129	135	143
61	132	138	146
62	135	141	149
63	138	144	152
64	141	147	155
65	144	150	158
66	147	153	161
67	150	156	164
68	153	159	167
69	156	162	170
70	159	165	173
71	161	168	176
72	164	171	179
73	167	174	182
74	170	177	185
75	173	180	188
76	176	183	191
77	179	186	194
78	182	189	197
79	185	191	200
80	188	193	203

WRIST GIRTH MEASUREMENTS		
BONE STRUCTURE (estimate)	**WOMEN** (inches)	**MEN** (inches)
Low	5¼ and below	6¼ and below
Medium	5½–6	6¼–7
High	6 and up	7 and up

IDEAL WEIGHTS FOR WOMEN
Based on 18% Body Fat
and Degree of Muscularity

HEIGHT (inches)	DEGREE OF MUSCULARITY		
	Low	Medium	High
56	78	84	90
57	82	88	94
58	86	92	98
59	90	96	102
60	94	100	106
61	98	104	110
62	102	108	114
63	106	112	118
64	110	116	122
65	114	120	126
66	118	124	130
67	122	128	134
68	126	132	138
69	130	136	142
70	134	140	146
71	138	144	150
72	142	148	154
73	146	152	158
74	150	156	162
75	154	160	166
76	158	164	170

reasonable alternative. However, if you have an opportunity to be tested at a fitness center or clinic by experienced and qualified personnel, then we recommend you get them to determine your percentage of fat and desired weight.

A body fat classification chart is presented in the table below. Although the norms reflect percentages for young men and women, we feel confident that they represent reasonable guides for self-evaluations regardless of age. We should point out that a normal rating refers to an average of the ratings of all the people we have measured. This does not necessarily mean this is the most desired rating for you. A body fat between 10 and 12% of total body weight is considered excellent for the men; by contrast, 18 to 20% body fat for women is considered excellent and generally signifies trimness. Over 25% body fat in men and over 30% in women indicates obesity — too much fat.

BODY FAT NORMS

CLASSIFICATION	WOMAN (%)	MEN (%)
Very low fat: skinny	14.0-16.9	7.0-9.9
Low fat: trim	17.0-19.9	10.0-12.9
Average fat: normal	20.0-23.9	13.0-16.9
Above normal fat: plump	24.0-26.9	17.0-19.9
Very high fat: fat	27.0-29.9	20.0-24.9
Obese: over fat	30.0 and higher	25.0 and higher

Body proportions. Regardless of weight, a body with proper proportions will look better. So what are proper proportions for women? What are proper proportions for men? And how do you rate? Along with knowing your body fat percentage and your ideal weight, measuring the girth of certain parts of the body will further indicate the trimness of your body. Such insight will help you set reasonable goals for yourself.

You need a friend or your spouse to help measure your body girths, a measuring tape (one made of fiberglass is preferred), and a piece of paper or an index card to record your measurements. You should stand tall and relaxed while being measured. The tape should be applied with even pressure (not too tightly) without compressing the underlying tissue. Take the measurements at the sites listed in the next chart.

SITES FOR MEASUREMENTS

Chest. At the nipple line and at the midpoint of a normal breath.

Waist. At the minimal abdominal girth, below the rib cage and just above the top of the hip bone.

Hips. At the level of the symphisis pubis in front, at the maximal protrusion of the buttocks in back. Be sure your feet are together when measuring this circumference.

Thigh. At the crotch level and just below the fold of the buttocks (gluteal fold).

Calf. At the maximal circumference.

Ankle: At the minimal circumference, usually just above the ankle bones.

Upper Arm. At the maximal circumference; with arm extended, palm up.

Wrist. At the most minimal circumference; with arm extended, palm up.

The following lists give recommended girth proportions for women and men. These serve only as a general reference based on measurements of many people who we would classify as trim and well proportioned. Record your measurements.

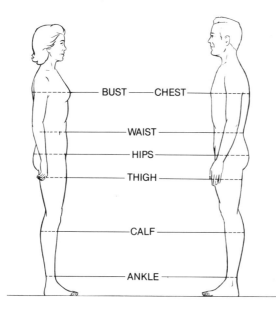

Recommended Girth Proportions for Women:

	Your Measurements
Bust should measure same as hips.	_____ inches
Waist should measure 10 inches less than bust or hips.	_____
Hips should measure same as bust.	_____
Thighs should measure 6 inches less than waist.	_____
Calves should measure 6 to 7 inches less than thighs.	_____
Ankles should measure 5 to 6 inches less than calves.	_____
Upper arm should measure twice the size of the wrist.	_____

Recommended Girth Proportions for Men:

	Your Measurements
Chest should measure same as hips.	_____ inches
Waist should measure 5 to 7 inches less than chest or hips.	_____
Hips should measure same as chest.	_____
Thighs should measure 8 to 10 inches less than waist.	_____
Calves should measure 7 to 8 inches less than thighs.	_____
Ankles should measure 6 to 7 inches less than calves.	_____
Upper arm should measure twice the size of the wrist.	_____

Measuring Your Muscular Strength and Endurance

Muscular strength, the ability to apply force, and muscular endurance, the capacity to exert force (strength) repeatedly over a period of time, are basic elements of physical fitness. However, to suggest definite strength or muscular endurance goals is questionable. Body build (weight, height, fatness) and anatomical differences can greatly affect one's performance on physical tests purporting to measure strength and muscular endurance. Nevertheless, it is worthwhile to appraise the strength and endurance of your muscles.

Obviously, to be effective in everyday tasks and to participate in our favorite recreational sports we don't need the muscle power of the top athlete. But some strength is needed. Furthermore, lower back pain, a common complaint of many men and women, has been linked to muscular weakness. Appropriate exercises can help eliminate such pain.

Our aim here is to help you assess your strength and muscular endurance so that you can determine whether they are adequate for everyday living and leisure activities. In Chaper 13 you'll find suggestions for developing and maintaining strength and muscular endurance. The self-testing presented in the following section will provide reasonable estimates of overall body strength and endurance capabilities. With this insight about your weaknesses and strengths, you will be able to set goals and arrange a program for toning your muscles to sustain the rigors of an active lifestyle.

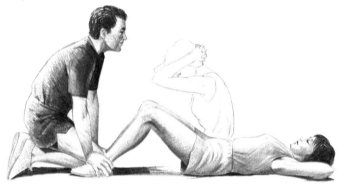

Figure 11. The sit-up test.

The sit-up test (bent knee). The sit-up test in Figure 11 has been used extensively for years to determine the strength and endurance of the abdominal muscles. Lie on your back, feet under a firm support (a friend may hold your feet) with knees bent at approximately 90°, feet flat on the floor, and hands interlocked behind your head. A full sit-up is counted when you have curled your back and raised your trunk until your lower back is at least perpendicular to the floor and then returned to the starting position. The total number of sit-ups performed in 60 seconds is your score for this test. Don't be discouraged if it's a struggle to do just one. This is a common occurrence with beginners in our program. Again, Chapter 13 shows you how to strengthen your abdominal muscles.

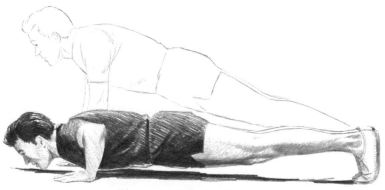

Figure 12. The push-up test.

The Push-Up Test. The push-up (Figure 12) is another test that has been used extensively for measuring the strength and endurance of the muscles in the upper body. (*Caution:* if you have a heart problem, do not take this test without a physician's permission.) Start in a front-leaning rest position, supporting your body on your hands and toes. Lower your body by bending at the elbows until your chest touches the floor. Keep your body flat and rigid. Return to the starting position. Your score is the number of correct complete push-ups you can do. Don't despair if you can't do even one push-up. Chapter 13 shows how to modify this exercise so you can gradually and sensibly improve the strength and endurance of your upper body muscles.

The table below presents some muscular endurance standards based on our observations of both men and women. It is quite common, especially for older people who have been inactive, not to do well on these tests. However, by including a few special exercises in each workout, you will gradually be able to improve your strength and muscular endurance.

MUSCULAR STRENGTH AND ENDURANCE STANDARDS FOR ADULT MEN AND WOMEN	
Sit-ups (60 seconds)	Push-ups (front leaning position)
Excellent 30 or more	15 or more
Good 25 to 29	10 to 14
Fair 20 to 24	5 to 9
Poor less than 20	less than 4

Measuring Your Flexibility

Flexibility is the ability to use a muscle throughout its maximum range of motion. The loss of the ability to bend, twist, and stretch results from muscle disuse, such as in excessive periods of sitting or standing. Sedentary living habits can lead to shortened muscles and tendons, lower back pain, and an imbalance of strength between opposing pairs of muscles. The shortening of the hamstrings (muscles located in the back of the thighs) is a very common disorder. The loss of flexibility limits your ability to walk smoothly, to sit down or stand up gracefully, and to perform efficiently in recreational pursuits. Extreme flexibility, however, has no advantage. If your joints are too loose or flexible, you may become more susceptible to injuries of the joints. Exercises for stretching the major muscle groups are recommended in Chapter 7. Although no single test will provide adequate information about the flexibility of all the major joints of the body, the following trunk flexion test provides a reasonable indication of your ability to stretch.

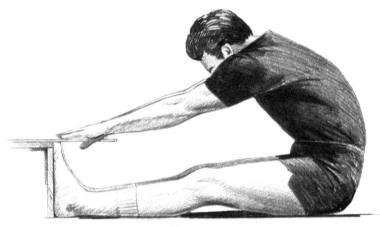

Figure 13. The trunk flexion test.

Trunk flexion test. The purpose of this test is to measure your ability to bend your trunk and to stretch the muscles of the back and the back thigh muscles (hamstrings). Sit with your legs fully extended and the bottom of your feet flat against a box projecting from the wall. See Figure 13. Now bend your trunk while extending (stretching) your arms and hands forward as far as possible and hold for a count of three. With a ruler, have your spouse or a friend measure (in inches) the distance before or beyond the edge of the box that you reach. Distances before the edge (not able to reach your toes) are expressed in negative scores; those beyond the edge are expressed as positive scores. The table below gives standards for flexibility. Regular performance of the battery of stretching exercises suggested in Chapter 7 will help you become more flexible in all parts of your body.

STANDARDS FOR SIT AND REACH TEST

	WOMEN	MEN
Normal range	-4 to $+10$ in.	-6 to $+8$ in.
Average values	$+2$ in.	$+1$ in.
Desired range	$+2$ to $+6$ in.	$+1$ to $+5$ in.

A Final Word On Self-Testing

The self-tests suggested in this chapter are easily administered and can be successfully used for rating your physical fitness. Care and accuracy are important when taking these tests. You are only fooling yourself if you do not perform the tests properly and record your true scores.

Now that you have a fairly good idea of how you stack up, I hope you have the incentive to set up a personal program of exercise. Knowing your physical fitness status will assist you in establishing a beginning point in your program. If you are still in doubt about your state of physical fitness, begin your program at the lowest level. You can always adjust upward.

As you progress with your program, retest yourself from time to time. Use the following personal fitness profile record to track your progress. Be sure to set reasonable goals. It will be gratifying when you begin to see favorable changes and improvements. Although testing should not dominate your exercise program, it can be a worthwhile motivator to greater effort and to regular exercise habits.

PERSONAL FITNESS PROFILE RECORD

	NOW Date:	3 MONTHS Date:	6 MONTHS Date:	1 YEAR Date:	2 YEARS Date:	3 YEARS Date:
Sitting Heart Rate (bts/min)						
Blood Pressure (mm/Hg)						
Body Weight						
% Body Fat						
Maximal Oxygen Uptake						
Maximal MET Level						
Distance Run (time to run 1.5 to 2 miles)						
Sit-Ups (no./min)						
Push-Ups (no.)						
Sit and Reach (in.)						

Summary

In this chapter I attempted to provide you with all the essentials for having your fitness status evaluated. These recommendations are based on the most current state of the art for fitness evaluation. If you are getting along in years (over 35) and have been inactive recently, then you should strongly consider a medical evaluation that includes at least a twelve-lead electrocardiogram and blood pressure. A graded exercise test on a treadmill or bicycle ergometer with monitored electrocardiogram is highly recommended. A blood profile and body composition are additional measures that are helpful to have but not as necessary. Limited availability of qualified health personnel and facilities may make it difficult for you to comply with these recommendations.

The inability to be exercise-tested doesn't mean you cannot participate in a program. It does, however, necessitate that you use good discretion. With the help of your family physician and the self-testing guidelines in this chapter you have the ingredients for evaluating your present condition. The fitness level table on pages 78, 79 has been developed to assist you in determining a proper place for starting your workouts. I must emphasize that you should use good judgement and not try to do too much, too soon. Careful adherence to the suggestions in this chapter will do much for carrying out a safe and effective physical fitness program. Use the chart at the end of this chapter for recording your fitness measurements so you can keep track of your training progress.

chapter six

Getting Ready—Some General Considerations

I hope that you have determined your current level of fitness and want to become more physically fit. Now I want to begin showing you how to accomplish this goal. I will get more specific and help you select a program that best fits your needs.

The next chapter will show you how to warm up properly with a series of stretching exercises. Chapters 8 through 12 present continuous, rhythmic endurance-type activities that were selected because they are the best modes for you to develop to the utmost your cardiorespiratory system. Along with detailed explanations on each endurance-type activity, a series of sequentially arranged workouts are provided. These workouts have been developed over the years and used to help people of all ages reach their physical potentials.

If you are overweight, have been inactive, or if you are over 40, walking is probably your best choice for starting a program. For sure, it is your safest form of exercise. A little caution at the beginning will make your initial efforts more comfortable. Many people encounter ligament or joint problems of the legs if they begin with a program of running. For this reason, a regulated program of walking geared to gradual increases in distance and vigor is one of the most suitable ways for beginning a fitness program. Once you can walk three miles briskly and your body has adjusted to this effort, you are ready for a more strenuous endeavor such as short periods of running alternated with walking. So, if you have been inactive, I recommend you start with the walking program in Chapter 8, even if you scored well on the tolerance test.

Walking—and for the more physically active, running—are the simplest activities for beginning an exercise program. These are the modes I have used the most over the past 20 years for getting people started. The fundamental advantage of these two activities is the ease with which they meet individual needs, regardless of age, sex, or level of fitness. But activities other than walking and running can be readily employed as suitable conditioners. For this reason programs for both bicycling and swimming have been developed in case you prefer them. All four modes can be utilized to provide an adequate workload for developing cardiorespiratory fitness. After a good warm-up, the choice is yours. Just remember to apply the basics of training (intensity, duration, and frequency, as recommended in Chapter 4) to produce a training effect regardless of the activity you choose.

Chapters, 8, 9, 10, and 11 can help you construct your own conditioning program using any or all of the four basic modes. Chapter 14 can help you establish an effective weight control program involving your exercise activities. Chapter 13 provides the basics for those desiring to develop and maintain muscular strength and endurance. Chapter 12 provides information on aerobic dance and how to use indoor fitness equipment properly. In Chapter 15, a wide variety of sports and popular activities, such as racquetball and roller skating, are evaluated for their worth as fitness developers.

General Considerations in Establishing Your Fitness Program

Before going to the next chapters, I want to give you some general advice that may help you structure your fitness program more effectively. Although each activity has its own specific characteristics, certain suggestions apply to all. Here are some:

Make It Personal

Keep in mind as you establish and follow your plan of exercise that *you can never begin too low in the charts, and the steps you take can never be too small!* Your present level of fitness is the key factor for determining a safe starting point. Don't worry about keeping up or catching up with your friends and neighbors. Don't let your ego push you beyond what's practical for you. Remember, your goal is to live at *your* fullest physical potential.

Proceed Gradually

My experience clearly indicates that most people want to do too much, too soon. A common notion is that if it doesn't hurt, it can't be effective. Don't believe it! Don't force yourself to suffer. My approach to exercise training is to stay well within each person's capabilities but at an intensity that is sufficient for favorable physical improvement. This is why I use the target heart rate and suggest that you stay close to it. If you exercise at too high a level of intensity, your workout becomes drudgery, and you might become discouraged.

Remember, this is a lifetime pursuit. I don't want you to get discouraged and quit after a few days or weeks. In all of these activities your exercise pulse rate will be used for regulating the intensity. Exercising at a training heart rate near 75% of the range between your resting and maximal heart rates is the recommended target for providing a proper exercise stimulus to your body. It may not be wise or possible for some of you to reach your target during your early stages of training. Don't despair! As you work your way through the charts you will become more fit and can easily sustain a workout at your target rate.

Although some of the charts refer to distances covered, your main concern in the beginning should be to sustain vigorous movement over a sufficient period of time in order to create a training effect. Knowing the distance helps, but during the initial weeks of your program you should not be concerned with trying to cover a distance as fast as you can. In other words, don't make it a race each day. Later, you may set goals to pick up your tempo, but no workout should be an all-out effort. Any reference to distance is there only to help you gauge your pace. We want you to be persistent *and* reasonable. Proceed gradually!

Set Reasonable Goals

Each exercise chart in this book represents a series of goals that can be reached in every workout. If you select a realistic starting point, the step-by-step increases built into the charts will give you reasonable goals in the initial months of your training. After you have worked your way through these planned progressions, you will be ready to assume the responsibility for creating your own workouts.

Although we provide carefully planned workouts, we encourage you to set some additional personal goals. For example, walkers may want to set a goal to eventually walk for one hour. Later, your goal may be to cover four miles in an hour. A common goal for runners is to complete that first mile, and then to complete two miles without stopping. Swimmers and cyclists can easily set similar goals for time or distance. The feeling of personal satisfaction that comes from reaching such goals will reinforce your will to keep going.

Keep a Record

After completing each workout, check it off on the chart you are following. Most of us keep a daily record of our workouts. I never did this until a few years ago when a friend gave me a runner's calendar. After realizing the value of the records, I now encourage others to keep track of their workouts. Whether you walk, run, swim, or cycle for fitness, posting your total mileage or the time spent during each workout provides a reinforcement on what you have accomplished. For now, you can rate your progress by checking off the charts provided in this book.

Coping With the Weather

Working out in inclement weather can be invigorating provided you use good judgment. You may enjoy working out in the rain, but it would not be wise to work out in a downpour or a thunderstorm.

Cold weather workouts are fine if you dress properly. Frostbite can be a dangerous consequence of cold-weather activity, especially when it's colder than 20° F. You may even need to confine your workouts to an indoor facility on very cold days. Heart patients especially, should avoid extended exposure to the cold. Walking, running, and cycling are more complicated during the winter than during the warmer months. However, as you become acclimated to the conditions, the exhiliration experienced when exercising in the cold and snow helps to overcome the adversities of winter weather.

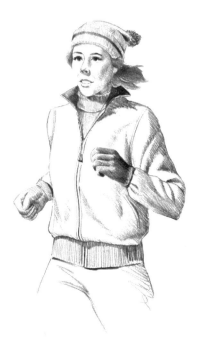

Workouts should probably be avoided during the hot and humid midday heat. In the warm months, however, an early-morning workout can be invigorating. Top off your sunrise workout with a relaxing shower and a balanced breakfast, and you are ready for a productive day. Swimming may be your best mode of exercise during hot and humid weather.

Doing Without Special Exercise Equipment

You don't need special exercise equipment to be fit. You can, however, exercise in your home by pedaling an exercise bike, walking or running on a treadmill, stepping up and down on the stepbench, crawling on a specially designed apparatus, or rowing a machine. These are possible alternatives for people who are either self-conscious about getting outside or who are restricted because they live in urban areas. See Chapter 12 on how to properly use indoor equipment. When the weather hinders outdoor activities or when a pool, track, or exercise area is not readily available, such indoor activities may be good substitutes for a day or so. However, you must be highly motivated to workout at home on a regular basis. Many people find bench stepping, stair climbing, or crawling-on-the-floor movements unnatural and boring. The end result is that they quit. There are better and more enjoyable ways to keep in shape. Remember, if exercise is to be a way of life, it must be an enjoyable and natural part of your day.

Most sport and athletic clubs have several types of expensive apparatus. Such layouts are quite impressive, but most of the apparatus is used for improving strength. The Universal and Nautilus systems are the two most commonly found in these centers. No question about it, these systems and others will give all the muscles of your body a good workout. But they cannot provide an adequate cardiorespiratory stimulus for improving your oxygen uptake capacity and overall circulation. This type of exercise will elevate your heart rate, but because of the straining of muscle groups against a resistance, your blood pressure can be elevated to a dangerous level. That is not the way to begin an exercise program. Anyone with heart disease or who is under-exercised should be discouraged from working out with such equipment at the beginning of a conditioning program. Get your heart in shape by walking, running, swimming, or cycling. Once you have progressed favorably (by completing our charts), then you may consider using these machines.

I recommend that you look with suspicion at exercise gadgets that promise total fitness; most are ineffective and just ways for a promoter to make money. I recall speaking in the Indianapolis area at a service club a few years ago. I was setting up my slide projector when one member of the group came up to me and said, "You must be the speaker." I acknowledged that I was and told him that my topic was physical fitness. His response was, "What kind of equipment are you selling?" It was an obvious question since service clubs are lucrative targets for fast-talking so-called fitness experts who sell special devices for executives to carry around in their attache cases. This incident provided my opening comment of the talk: "I want to assure you at the outset that my purpose here today is not to sell any kind of fitness gadget. In fact, you brought with you today the only equipment you need to get in shape and stay fit. You're sitting on it. It's your body! It may be a little rusty and bursting at the seams, but with some effort you can tune up this physiological wonder without any special equipment."

Most people think there is a magic piece of equipment yet to be discovered that will provide instant fitness without effort. To be fit, you don't need to use mechanical equipment, but you do need to use your physiological equipment.

Finding a Place to Work Out

In the chapters that follow we will be more specific about where to work out for each activity. Nevertheless, certain considerations are basic to all activities and need to be discussed at this point.

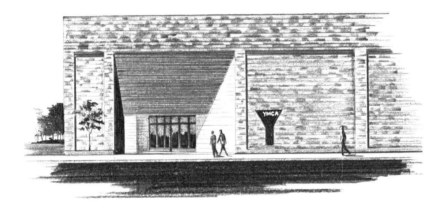

Joining an organized club or program. When you pay to exercise in facilities such as the YW/YMCA, community clubs, and fitness centers, the incentive to hang in there is greater. In addition, the company of others pursuing similar goals helps in the early stages of your fitness development. Such facilities provide a walking-running area or a swimming pool, plus additional exercise opportunities that are helpful for getting in shape. The possibility of getting good instruction and supervision, if you desire, is another benefit in these communal settings.

If you are interested in such places, be sure to choose one that has an honest commitment to the value of exercise. If they don't have adequate running and walking areas, be suspicious of their intentions. Don't be fooled by a roomful of expensive shiny machines with mirrors and carpeting. There is more to physical fitness than pushing weights or sitting in a jacuzzi or sauna. These mechanisms and baths are nice as long as proper areas for cardiorespiratory exercises are provided. So check for a track, a pool, and exercise bikes. If they have a preponderence of effortless machines that promise to vibrate or melt away unwanted inches, my advice is save your money and look elsewhere.

Check out the qualifications of the instructors and managers of these facilities. Are they qualified? Ask the instructors about their personal exercise habits. Do they run, swim, or cycle? What types of cardiorespiratory training do they promote?

Many people don't need to belong to a club or center. Actually, the material found in this book is all you need. If you desire company, then we suggest you find a friend or friends and use the guidelines suggested here.

Discovering alternatives. You do need a place to exercise. If you do not have an exercise facility to go to, then what are your alternatives? For many, your exercise facility is right outside your door. However, for those who live in cities or have to travel frequently, finding a place to exercise can be a problem.

There are parks, malls, parking lots, streets, and yards where you can walk and run. Safety might be a problem in some areas. Not only must you be concerned about cars and, in some places, muggers, but dogs can certainly interrupt a well-intended workout. However, as I've traveled around the country, I've always managed to find places to work out. In fact, it has become a challenge for me to find many different settings for my walking and running. For instance, I've run down Bourbon Street in New Orleans in the early morning hours, in the Disneyland parking lot at night, through downtown Seattle (hills and all), on the beaches of Maine, in the forests of Wisconsin and Michigan, in many hotel parking lots, and even in a few parking garages in snowy weather.

For some, these suggestions may seem impractical. Perhaps you don't want to be seen bouncing through your own neighborhood. If you don't want to let your neighbors in on your new adventure, consider walking or even driving to a nearby park, hotel parking lot, or a local schoolyard. Many people walk and run in the darkness or early morning hours to avoid revealing their intentions to friends and neighbors. In Muncie, we have installed a lighted half-mile running loop around the Human Performance Laboratory so that people can use this for walking and running at all hours of the day and night. It is not uncommon to see people travel from across town to use it. Why? Because it's safe, no one will laugh at them, and it offers the company of others. Hopefully, you can find similar areas that are suitable for you to maintain a regular and enjoyable exercise program. If you want to stay fit, you can find a way.

Dressing for the activity. Proper clothing is an important consideration. If swimming is your mode of working out, obviously you need only a bathing suit and an open swimming lane. However, aside from special uniforms and facilities that are appropriate for a particular sport, there are some general considerations for dressing properly for the occasion.

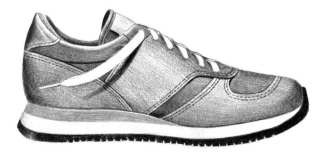

For running and other athletic activities, proper shoes are a must. The training shoe used by most runners is also recommended for walking. There are many fine training shoes on the market today with good multilayered sponge-like soles and strong heel counter. But some companies are now making so-called running shoes that sell at bargain prices. Many of these are of poor quality, and everything from blisters to shin splints may be part of the bargain. Buy quality shoes from a reputable sporting goods store. See Appendix B for more detailed explanation about the selection and proper fit of shoes for walking and running. Proper footwear is a wise investment. Special shoes are also made for other sports, such as tennis, hiking, and basketball; again, quality purchases are a must.

Your clothing should be light and loose-fitting. Cotton shorts and a T-shirt or blouse are adequate in warm weather. Nylon clothing should be avoided in the heat. Warm-up shirts and pants are all right too, but don't wear them during hot weather. Avoid the rubberized weight-reduction outfits. These only keep your body heat in and produce sweat; they do not help you lose body fat and can be very dangerous in hot and humid weather.

Men should wear an athletic supporter or jockey-type shorts; regular undershorts will do for women. An essential part of the female's ensemble is the bra. Sportswear companies now cater to the active sportswomen. When selecting a bra for exercising activity, choose one that has no chafing points such as metal fasteners, hooks, or wires. The ideal bra doesn't have seams, is made of soft cotton, and can be pulled on over the head (an all-stretch type). It must provide enough support to restrict bouncing to a comfortable level.

One pair of light cotton or wool socks are recommended for walking, running, and cycling. Wearing two pairs of socks (one of them thin) is necessary only when the activity involves shifting movements, as in racquetball or tennis. Many find the anklets quite suitable.

If you run or walk in the winter cold, be sure to wear thermal mittens and a stocking cap or wool ski mask. Keep your chest and rib cage warm with several thin layers, one of them a turtleneck shirt. For example, wear a T-shirt, a long-sleeve turtleneck, another T-shirt, and, when needed, a nylon windbreaker with a zippered front. Winter walking and running can be enjoyable and safe if you dress properly. Later chapters will cover the specifics for each activity in more detail.

Working Out With Others

Most of us enjoy doing things with others—going to the theater, ball games, picnics. Much of the fun from these outings comes from doing them with friends or relatives. So why not plan your workouts with friends or relatives who have fitness capacities and activity interests similar to yours? Make it a recreation period of social fun.

For many men and women, exercising with others has been a key factor in maintaining the fitness habit, especially in the early stages of a group program. Of course in the end you must provide your own impetus and motivation to keep up a regular program. Once you experience the fun, relaxation, and exihilaration that comes with each workout, you will not need the prodding of others to keep in shape. Instead, you will exercise because you want to and because you enjoy the total body stimulus exercise provides. The company of friends then becomes a bonus for your fitness workouts.

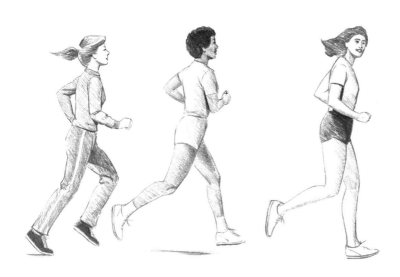

Avoiding Injury

During the early stages of an exercise program, the chance of injury to the muscles, joints, or ligaments is quite high. It takes time for your muscles and joints to adjust to the stress of exercise. We cannot stress it strongly enough: *Do not hurry your fitness program.* Prolonged fatigue for an hour or more after your workout means your program is too demanding. Avoid exhaustion. Your exercise should leave you with a sense of pleasant relaxation and well-being. Generally, it isn't a lack of "wind" that slows up beginning training programs, but injured joints and muscles.

Be injury-conscious in the early weeks of your fitness workouts and try to avoid unnecessary muscle soreness and injury. An injury that limits or completely terminates your regular workouts can be very discouraging. Staying injury-conscious is a preventive measure that can help make your liftime commitment to fitness safe and pleasurable.

Using the Charts

The exercise charts for walking, running, cycling, and swimming have been developed from our knowledge and actual experience in starting people on a conditioning program. They are designed to assist you in a step-by-step manner through the early stages of training.

Using the charts properly will help you set attainable goals. Each step in the charts has been planned so that you can complete each exercise session. Such success will reinforce your continuous participation. If you are not achieving these goals on a regular basis, then you are probably over-estimating your capabilities and not evaluating the situation realistically. Be honest with yourself. The charts are only guidelines for your participation. They are not objectives etched in stone to be reached at all costs. Reassessments and adjustments may be necessary as you proceed with your program. Just keep in mind that your ultimate goal is being fit; living at *your* fullest physical potential.

chapter seven

Stretching for Flexibility

For many people, the thought of calisthenics brings back images of tedious, boring, and maybe senseless routines from gym classes or athletic practices. The military approach (exercises in strict cadence) has never been popular. Nevertheless, a well-rounded physical fitness program needs a segment of calisthenic-type exercises.

Warm-up exercises not only stretch the muscles for the ensuing workout but gradually prepare the cardiorespiratory system for the main workout.

It must be emphasized that the exercises presented in this chapter do not comprise a total program of fitness. A cardiorespiratory endurance activity must be your main conditioning bout with these exercises serving as supplements. Cardiorespiratory endurance-type exercise (see following chapters) such as brisk walking, running, cycling, and swimming provide the needed total body involvement required to stimulate your heart and circulatory system. In general, calisthenic exercises do not provide such a stimulus to the heart and lungs.

Many people do calisthenic-type exercises in hopes of trimming unwanted inches off their waists or hips. Despite what many so-called exercise specialists claim, there is no concrete evidence that exercising a particular spot of the body will take off inches. Inches will slowly come off at the fatty sites when the body's metabolic rate is increased substantially on a regular basis. Doing calisthenics to firm up muscle groups is a reasonable objective, but trying to lose inches of fat with spot reducing exercises doesn't work.

Unfortunately many men and women believe that physical fitness is reflected only in external appearance. They have the mistaken notion that if you look fit, you are fit. Few people realize that a trim and firm body, a radiant complexion, and youthful vigor come not only from exercise that improves muscle tone, but also from activities that stress the circulatory and respiratory systems. Physical fitness, with the extra benefits of fat loss and improved body proportions, require a vigorous stimulation of the heart, lungs, and muscles. Stretching exercises or calisthenics are just one part of a total conditioning program.

The Basic Twelve

The selection of exercises that follow can easily be incorporated into your fitness program. The Basic Twelve provide a means of loosening, stretching, shaping, and strengthening your major muscle groups. They were developed after several years of experimenting and now represent the basic warm-ups we use in the Ball State Fitness Program.

You may already have a series of exercises that you do on a regular basis. Most likely they are quite similar to the ones we are about to recommend. There's no reason to stop doing them and start doing ours as long as they are stretching and toning most of your major muscle groups.

This sequence of exercises is a combination of conventional, as well as some of the newer yoga-type, calisthenic exercises. Yoga involves holding a static position (posture) for a period of time. Such a posture puts the muscles and connective tissues being stretched at their greatest possible length. Static stretching (as this method is often called) has proved very effective. Bouncy movements while exercising impose sudden strains on the muscles involved and such bobbing causes reflexes that actually oppose the desired stretching. Therefore, it's not wise to bob and bounce while doing the exercises. Instead, stretch slowly, being careful to stretch the muscles to a point of tension where there is a slight to moderate discomfort. Overstretching, especially if done with rapid movements, can lead to injury.

Many of the leg-stretching exercises should be repeated after your main exercise bout. These should be done routinely during the cooldown phase of your workout. Walking, cycling, and especially running rate low in flexibility development. In fact, daily running can even have some bad effects on the muscles of the legs. Quite often, runners experience an abnormal tightening of the back muscles of the thigh (hamstrings). This can lead to strength imbalances, causing injuries. The running muscles, especially the muscles in the back of your legs, need to be stretched before and after each workout. Distance running requires a relatively small range of movements, and when the leg muscles are used repeatedly over a sustained period of time, they tend to become very tight. Thus, there is a definite need to stretch the large leg muscles regularly.

Although these exercises were primarily developed for stretching before and after a conditioning workout, we suggest you constantly "think stretching." We encourage the participants in our program to stretch whenever they get a chance, any time during the day. Once you become familiar with the main muscles that need stretching, you can easily do some of the exercises as you stand or sit, any time during the day. They may help you avoid tight muscles and may even refresh you.

Before doing the warm-ups we recommend that you walk for a few minutes. This gets your heart pumping and blood flowing. This is especially wise before beginning an early morning workout. During the day, after you have been up and around, the need for preliminary walking prior to doing the exercises is not as necessary.

On the following pages you will find instructions for the Basic Twelve. (A short form, the Quick Six, is suggested later.) Do these stretching exercises at a tempo that suits you. They are presented in a progressive sequence that's easy to follow: four standing up, four lying down, four standing up.

The purpose of each exercise is given. The starting position is described, and the proper instructions are presented, along with illustrations for movement. Three levels of exertion (light, moderate, heavy) are suggested for each activity, with the appropriate numbers of repetitions indicated within the circles. Start with the lightest level and work toward the moderate and heavy.

Remember as you exercise, avoid bobbing or forcing your body into unaccustomed positions. If you haven't been exercising regularly, it will take a while before you can stretch some of those tight muscles fully. Don't hurry. Proceed at a pace that's comfortable yet will gradually accomplish what you want — more flexibility.

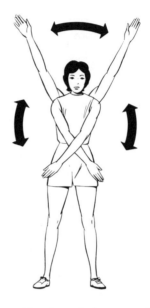

Figure 14a. Arm circles—cross body

1. ARM CIRCLES

Purpose:	To loosen and stretch the muscles of the arms and the shoulder region.
Starting Position:	Stand with your feet shoulder-width apart and your arms at your sides.
Movement:	In each of the four following exercises, your arms should make large, sweeping circles. Keep your elbows straight and swing your arms from the shoulders.
Inward Cross-Body:	Swing your arms inward, upward, and around crossing in front of the face and body.

(10)   (15)   (20)

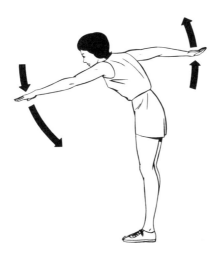

Figure 14b. Arm circles—forward.

Outward Cross Body:	Swing your arms outward, upward, and around, crossing in front of your body.

(10)   (15)   (20)

Forward:	Swing your arms forward (as in a crawl swimming motion), making large sweeping circles. Count a complete circle with the left *and* right arm as one revolution.

(10)   (15)   (20)

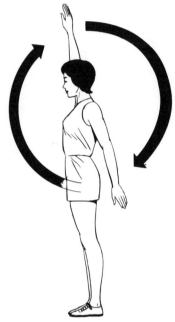

Figure 14c. Arm circles—backward.

Backward: Swing your arms backward (as in a backward swimming crawl), making large
sweeping circles.

Note: Start with the lightest exertion (first circle) and as the weeks pass
you may wish to increase the intensity of your warm-up to a moderate
level (middle circle) or a vigorous level (the third circle).

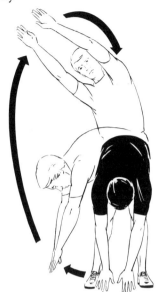

Figure 15. Trunk bender.

2. TRUNK BENDER

Purpose:	To stretch the leg muscles and low-back extensor muscles.
Starting Position:	Stand with your feet five to six inches apart and parallel to each other.
Movement:	Bend forward from the waist, allowing your arms, trunk, and head to hang freely. Reach to touch the floor, slowly. Then twist the trunk and reach for the outside of one shoe and slowly return to an upright position by coming up from the side. Again bend forward from the waist and alternate your movement to the other side. Repeat the exercise. Normally, your knees should be held straight; however, a slight bend does not hinder the effectiveness of the exercise so long as you feel a slight to moderate stretch discomfort in your rear leg muscles.

④   ⑥   ⑧

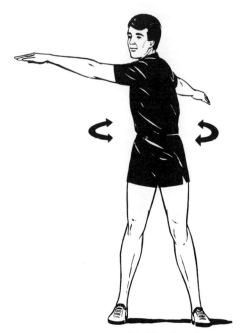

Figure 16. Trunk twister.

3. TRUNK TWISTER

Purpose: To loosen and stretch muscles in the
                       back, sides, and shoulder region.

Starting Position: Stand with your feet shoulder-width
                       apart, arms extended to the sides at
                       shoulder level.

Movement: While keeping your heels flat on the
                       floor, twist your trunk to the right slowly
                       as far as you can turn, then return to
                       starting position. Now twist slowly to the
                       left. Repeat the complete movement
                       slowly.

                            ⑥   ⑨   ⑫

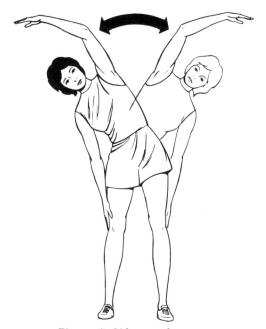

Figure 17. Side stretcher.

4. SIDE STRETCHER

Purpose:	To loosen and stretch the side muscles of the trunk.
Starting Position:	With your feet shoulder-width apart with one arm extended upward (palm facing inward) and the other arm extended downward (palm touching the side of your thigh).
Movement:	Bend your trunk to the side of the lower extended arm. Reach with your lower hand and stretch, sliding the hand down your thigh to the knee or lower. The other arm should be stretched over your head and in the direction of body's lean. Return to the starting position and repeat the exercise on the other side. Alternate.

$$\textcircled{6} \qquad \textcircled{9} \qquad \textcircled{12}$$

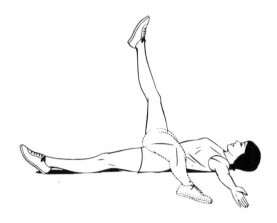

Figure 18. Leg-overs.

5. LEG-OVERS

Purpose:	To loosen and stretch the rotator muscles of the lower back and the pelvic region.
Starting Position:	Lie on your back with your legs extended, and your arms extended at shoulder level (palms up).
Movement:	Keep the knee extended as you raise your leg to a vertical position (point your toes). The opposite leg should remain on the floor in extended position; keep the back of that leg on the floor. While keeping your shoulders, arms, and back on the floor, reach with the vertically extended leg across your body to the extended opposite hand. Stretch to touch your toe to the floor in the area of the extended hand, then return your leg first to the vertical position and then to the floor. Follow the same procedure with the other leg. Repeat the complete exercise.

$$\textcircled{4} \qquad \textcircled{6} \qquad \textcircled{8}$$

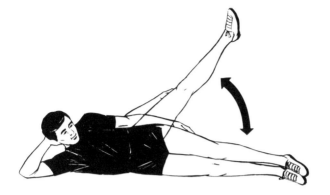

Figure 19. Side leg raises.

6. SIDE LEG RAISES

Purpose:	To strengthen and stretch the lateral hip muscles.
Starting Position:	Lie on your right side, in extended position, with your head resting on your right forearm and hand.
Movement:	Raise your left leg upward from the floor (keeping the knee extended and toes pointed away) to a position well above the horizontal, then return to starting position. Keep your pelvis perpendicular to the floor. After completing the repetitions for one side, repeat the exercise on the other side.

(10)   (15)   (20)

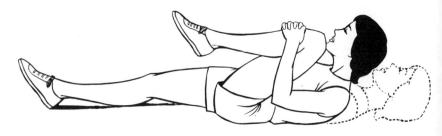

Figure 20. Low back and hip stretcher.

7. LOW-BACK STRETCHER

Purpose:	To stretch and loosen the lower back and hip flexor muscles.
Starting Position:	Lie on your back with knees straight.
Movement:	Pull one knee to your chest. Grasp the leg just below the knee and pull the knee toward your chest. Hold for five seconds. Then, curl your shoulders and head toward the knee. Hold for five or more seconds. Return to starting position and repeat exercise with other leg. Alternate.

(4)   (6)   (8)

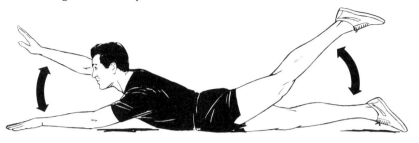

Figure 21. Arm and leg lifter.

8. ARM AND LEG LIFTER

Purpose:	To strengthen and stretch the extensor muscles of the back and hip.
Starting Position:	Lie face down (prone position) with your arms extended over your head and your legs extended.
Movement:	Raise your right arm and left leg simultaneously and keep them extended for a few seconds. Then return to starting position. Now raise the left arm and right leg simultaneously. Alternate. Do this exercise slowly; do not jerk your legs and arms.

(4)   (6)   (8)

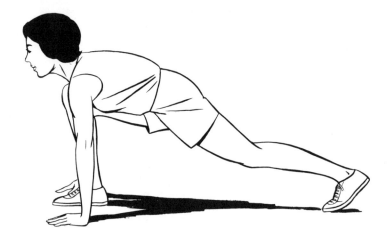

Figure 22a. Forward stride stretcher.

9. STRIDE STRETCHER, FORWARD AND LATERAL

a) Forward

Purpose:	To stretch the lower back muscles, hip flexors, and leg muscles.
Starting Position:	Move your leg forward so that it is flexed under your chest, knee directly over the ankle, and your other leg stretched out behind.
Movement:	With your hands on the floor and your forward heel on the floor, roll your body forward while pushing your hips down toward the floor. Hold for five or more seconds. Repeat the exercise with the other leg forward.

⑤   ⑩   ⑮

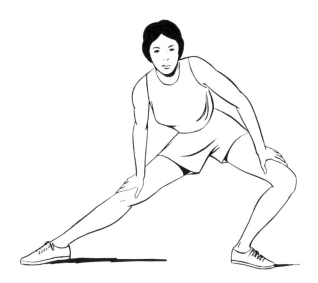

Figure 22b. Lateral stride stretcher.

b) Lateral

Purpose:	To stretch the inner sides of the leg muscles.
Starting Position:	Spread your legs in a wide straddle position, toes pointing straight ahead.
Movement:	Shift your weight sidewards so that most of your weight is on one leg. Hold this position for five seconds or more, feeling a moderate stretching discomfort on the inner muscles of the thigh. Then shift weight over to the other foot for the same interval of time. Repeat.

(4)   (6)   (8)

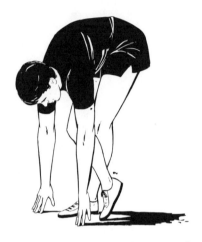

Figure 23a. Standing hamstring stretcher.

10. HAMSTRING STRETCHER, STANDING OR LEANING

a) Standing

Purpose:	To stretch the hamstring (large muscles on the back of the thigh) and lower back muscles.
Starting Position:	Stand and cross one leg in front of the other. The toes of the front leg should touch the floor, heel up.
Movement:	Slowly bend forward from the waist, keeping your rear leg straight (heel on floor). Try to stretch until you feel a slight discomfort in the muscles of your rear leg. Hold the position for five or more seconds and return to the starting position. Stretch the other leg in a similar manner. Repeat a few times.

②   ④   ⑥

Either a or b is sufficient for stretching the hamstring muscles.

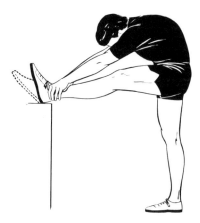

Figure 23b. Leaning hamstring stretcher.

b) Leaning

Purpose:	To stretch the hamstring muscles and lower back muscles.
Starting Position:	Raise one leg and rest the heel of the foot on a solid object such as a table or chair, toes pointing up.
Movement:	Reach and lean toward the raised foot until you feel an easy stretch and hold for a few seconds. While holding the stretch, you can also slowly roll the heel forward (pointed toes moving away) to an extended position; then slowly roll heel back, drawing toes as close as possible to your body. Be careful not to over-stretch. Repeat a few times and then stretch the other leg.

          (6)

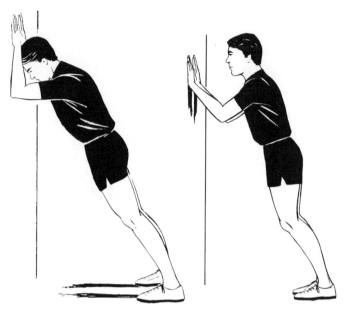

Figures 24a and b. Achilles and calf stretcher.

11. ACHILLES AND CALF STRETCHER*

Purpose:	To stretch the calf muscles and the heel cords (the achilles tendon).
Starting Position:	Stand facing a wall an arm's distance away, with your knees straight, toes slightly inward, and your heels flat on the floor.

Movement:

a. With hands resting on the wall, lean forward, bending your elbows slowly. Keep legs and body straight and heels on the floor. You will feel stretching discomfort in the calf and lower tendons attached to the heel. Hold for five or more seconds then return to the starting position.
b. Then, do the same exercise but bend the knees slightly and hold for five or more seconds before returning to starting position. This variation allows you to stretch an important muscle (the soleus) which lies directly under your calf muscle (gastrocnemius). Repeat each segment a few times.

*This exercise can also be done with one leg forward (knee bent) and the other leg back (knee straight). Alternate weight from leg to leg.

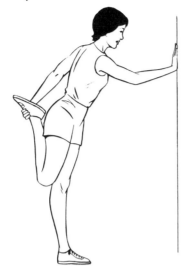

Figure 25. Standing quad stretcher.

12. STANDING QUAD STRETCHER

Purpose:	To stretch the quadriceps. Also expands chest and stretches shoulder muscles.
Starting Position:	While standing erect bend the right knee and lift the right foot directly behind the body. Hold the toes of the foot with the left hand. Use your right hand to balance on a wall or chair.
Movement:	Bend the lifted right knee and draw the leg up and back. Pull up the right leg until you feel a slight discomfort in the upper front thigh (quadricep muscles). Balance and hold firmly for five or more seconds. (It is important to stand erect while holding the stretch.) Repeat with the other leg.

$$\textcircled{2} \qquad \textcircled{4} \qquad \textcircled{6}$$

REMINDER: An easy way to remember the sequence of the BASIC TWELVE is four up (Exercises 1-4), four down (5-8), and 4 four up (9-12).

The Quick Six

The Basic Twelve are sound exercises that can be performed easily and safely. However, there are days when many of us are in a hurry and do not have the time or desire to do every exercise before working out. For those particular days we have identified six exercises that we feel *must* be done before each workout in order to avoid injury. We call them the Quick Six. They are as follows:

1. Trunk Bender
2. Side Stretcher
3. Stride Stretcher, Forward and Lateral
4. Achilles and Calf Stretcher
5. Hamstring Stretcher, Standing or Leaning
6. Standing Quad Stretcher

As you will note, all of these exercises can be performed without lying down. This makes them easy to remember (six up) and keeps you off the ground during inclement weather. However, most of your workouts should include the Basic Twelve.

Some Do's and Don'ts

1. Do warm up by doing stretching exercises before you workout (helps avoid injury).

2. Do follow the suggested sequence of exercises — for the Basic Twelve: four up, four down, four up, and for the Quick Six: six up (makes them easier to remember).

3. Do each exercise slowly and smoothly without jerking and bouncing (prevents injuries due to overstretching).

4. Do hold each stretching position for a few seconds (helps avoid jerking).

5. Don't strain. Go to the edge of your stretch until you feel a slight to moderate discomfort but stop before there is severe pain (helps avoid injury).

6. Do breathe deeply and rhythmically (helps you relax).

7. Do stretch after your workout and at other times during the day (keeps your body flexible).

SUMMARY

This chapter shows you good, sound, basic stretching exercises that are beneficial for muscle tone and flexibility. Once you learn the correct methods of performing these exercise movements you can easily make them a part of your regular routine.

Remember, stretching and toning exercises form just one phase of a complete physical fitness program. Despite what many people think, a program devoted exclusively to calisthenic-type exercises is not a satisfactory form of fitness exercise in itself. They do not provide adequate stimulation for the development of cardiorespiratory fitness. Instead, these basic calisthenic-type exercises serve as supplemental exercises for more vigorous types of exercise. They will help you warm up, stretch key muscle groups, and tone the major muscles of the body. When you combine these exercises with one of the cardiorespiratory endurance programs suggested in the following chapters and with one or more of your favorite sports, you will create a complete and highly effective activity program.

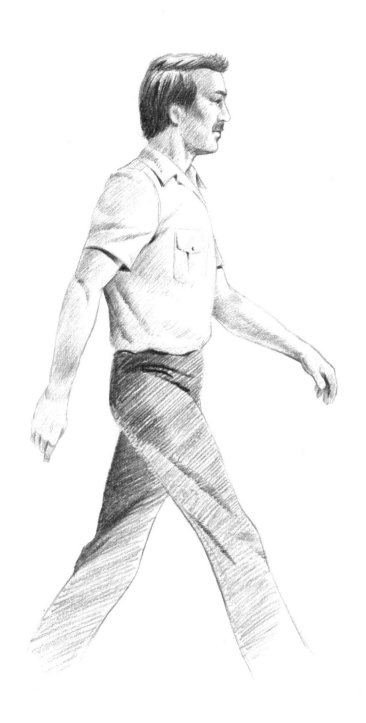

chapter eight

Walking

Walking is a natural and healthy form of exercise. Although less stressful than running, a brisk one-hour walk burns about 300 calories. We were designed to walk; even to walk incredible distances. Our ancestors at times made great migrations on foot, seeking a better life.

Many people think that walking is even better than running because walking does not place a heavy strain on the tendons of the foot and leg. Walkers endure far fewer injuries than runners.

For many people who want to get in shape, walking should be their first (and for many, their main) exercise activity. This is especially true for older people who have been inactive in recent years. Regardless of age, if you are extremely overweight, walking is your wisest choice. If you have been directed to this chapter because you presently have a low level of fitness (see Chapter 5), the suggestions that follow will help you improve your fitness so you can enjoy more strenuous activities. Forget about running until your body adjusts to sustained workouts of brisk walking on a regular basis, and you lose some weight (if you need to). You may not be able to run due to special medical limitations, or you just may not *want* to run.

Many people who want to get in shape do not want to run. In fact, they detest the thought of any form of jogging or running. Perhaps you fall into this category. Don't feel bad if you have such feelings. Believe it or not, some of our most avid runners started out as walkers. They had never done any exercise, so they assumed they wouldn't like it. But when they got into a regular program they began to feel better and decided to keep going.

Here are some common comments from regular walkers: "This program has helped me mentally as much as it has physically." "After my walking, I can go back home for a good hearty breakfast, and I'm ready to start the day on a positive basis." "I've been able to lose weight

133

and keep it off." "The most important thing I get from walking is *I feel better.*"

What Walking Can and Can't Do for You

Most injuries in beginning physical fitness programs are due to doing too much, too soon, too fast, too hard. In scientific studies, many people show improved physiological responses to endurance-type training programs, but injuries have often forced many people to interrupt or even stop their program. The exercise mode that most frequently causes such injuries is running. In contrast, walkers endure far fewer injuries than runners.

Recently, we studied 11 adults (average age 56) who took part in our brisk walking program. After 15 weeks in the program, the length of the exercise sessions had increased to as much as an hour and 15 minutes. The frequency of exercise sessions was no less than four times a week. I mention this to emphasize that *none* of the participants were forced to drop out because of an injury. Some of these people went on to a run-walk program after 15 weeks of walking. Some, either because of physical limitations or personal choice, are still walking on a regular basis. The few orthopedic problems of the legs and knees during this study were due to the fact that the walking provided a more tolerable working rate. In short, brisk walking proved invigorating for those older adults without being debilitating.

For many, a walk is a 15-minute stroll around the block. But it takes 15 minutes just to get going in a rhythmic stride. When I talk about fitness walking, I am talking about at least an hour of continuous and brisk walking at a pace that will stimulate the flow of blood in your body. You will not be able to accomplish this at first, but eventually your walking workout should be at that pace and duration. Because walking is lower in intensity (compared with running and swimming), it must be done longer if you are to reap significant fitness changes.

Several books have extolled the virtues of walking for physical fitness. I have personally reviewed these books, and I am sorry to report that many of them overstate the physiological benefits that come from fitness walking. Walking will improve circulation and lower your heart rate, but to state emphatically that it will do just as much for you as running is nonsense and cannot be substantiated with research. Some times these books are worded like running books with *walking* used in place of *running*. The honest enthusiasm for walking often gets out of hand.

Our aim is to show the way to live at your fullest physical potential, and walking may be the best mode of exercise for you. Or, it may be the pathway that will lead you to other exercise and sports accomplishments you had never thought possible.

Some Preliminary Considerations

The walking program is based on our experience with people who are at low levels of fitness. For most middle-aged and older people, especially those who are under-exercised, the walking charts are the safest and most appropriate guides to get a disciplined program going. Even if you feel capable of the effort, if you have been inactive in recent years, I highly recommend going slow at first and beginning a walking program.

Remember as you progress through the walking sessions, your first goal is to work up to a point where you can walk for a minimum of an hour. Then your goal is to cover as much distance as possible in an hour's time, keeping well within your physical capabilities. The charts are designed to help you progress gradually in this manner. You want to keep challenging your heart, enabling it to beat near your target heart rate. When you can briskly walk three miles with ease, you are ready for more vigorous activities.

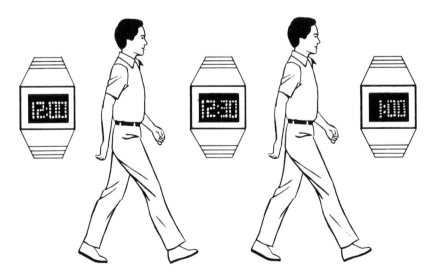

Before taking that first step, read the following suggestions on selecting a starting point, using the charts, how and where to walk, preventing injuries and taking your pulse to monitor the intensity of your workouts.

Selecting a Starting Point

You need to know your fitness level in order to determine a reasonable and safe starting point in your fitness walking program. If you took an exercise tolerance test and have a MET value you can easily determine your fitness level and starting point by referring to the table on pages 78 and 79. If you took our walking test, you have already determined an approximation of your maximal MET capacity and your starting point from this table. For example, if it took 25 minutes or more to walk a distance of one mile or if you were unable to complete the mile distance, your fitness level is very low and you must begin with the starter program (step 1) for walking and proceed accordingly. Let's say you were able to cover the mile in 22.5 minutes; you can skip the first two sessions (as the charts indicate) and begin at step 3 of the starter program. Those who are able to walk farther and faster will be able to start at a higher level.

As you walk you may find it difficult to reach your target heart rate. Don't despair! Because of the low intensity of walking, even briskly, it is difficult to reach your target rate. By gradually lengthening your duration and working toward a goal of one hour, you will compensate for the inability to raise your heart rate during the walking.

What to Wear

In Chapter 6, some general advice about what to wear when you work out is given. Nevertheless, its importance warrants including this topic again, especially in a more detailed manner.

Any activity in which there is an impact force applied to the feet, ankles, and knees can often cause some problems to the participant. The heavier you are, the greater the possibility of injuring the areas of the feet and lower legs. Of utmost importance then are the shoes you wear. Our experiences indicate that the running shoes on the market today are excellent shoes for walking. Such shoes have a good multi-layered sole, a strong heel counter, and a flexibile forefoot. Your canvas tennis sneakers won't do; neither will racquetball or basketball shoes.

Shoes of these types do not give enough of the special kind of support needed for running or walking briskly for an hour or more. When you look for a shoe store, find one that carries a variety of brands. One that specializes in running and athletic shoes is a safe bet. But be sure you try on more than one pair. Walk around in them. They should feel so good you can't wait to get going! For more information about shoes, turn to Appendix B, which gives suggestions for proper selection and fit.

Be sure to wear comfortable clothing. A general rule is to wear as little as you can. In hot, humid weather you want to wear clothing that fits loosely and is porous enough to allow your body to breathe. Cotton, or a combination of cotton and polyester, is your best bet. Cotton absorbs sweat and allows for evaporation of sweat easily. The key is not to trap heat or moisture. You want to avoid excessive dehydration, possible heat exhaustion, and heat stroke.

By contrast, in cold weather you want to trap the warm air coming off your body and hold it. Therefore, dress in layers. Keep the chest and rib cage warm with several thin layers, one shirt being a turtleneck. For example, wear a T-shirt, turtleneck, and a nylon windbreaker. Again, it depends on the conditions. Often people tend to overdress in the winter so the outer layer (windbreaker) should be easy to unzip and take off as your body warms. As you walk with the wind to your back you may need to zip open your jacket, but turning into the wind may require zipping up. Be sure to wear mittens and a stocking cap to keep the fingers and ears protected from frostbite. A cap also prevents you from losing valuable body heat. If you are still cold, add another layer of clothing, not heavier garments.

How To Walk

Walking for fitness takes special preparation. *You need to learn how to walk.* In the beginning, you should walk at a pace that is comfortable, natural, and rhythmic. Let your arms swing normally, in a relaxed (not forced) way. Stand tall with your head high. Let your heel hit first and roll on to the ball of your foot.

After a few walking sessions, your muscles and breathing will begin to adjust to the walking pace. You will be increasing your distance a little each day. Eventually, as you get in better shape, you can pick up your pace by striding out and walking faster. The idea is not to be breathless, but to be breathing faster and with greater depth than at rest. Your pace should always be challenging to your cardiorespiratory system.

This is why it is important to be aware of how close you are to your target heart rate. If during your walk you find it difficult to keep up the pace, we suggest that you slow down your walk for about a minute to recover before returning to your training pace. Alternating brisk walking with slower walking can allow you to sustain your workout and to accomplish your distance goal for that day.

Where To Walk

It's important to choose a good place to walk. By good, we mean a place with a stable and smooth surface. Rough and uneven surfaces may cause injury. Walk where it is safe, and if you walk at night or in the early morning darkness, always carry a flashlight. Avoid hills in the early stages of your training. It is always wise to avoid automobile traffic and the accompanying pollutants. Many people walk in shopping malls, enabling them to walk in all kinds of weather. But again, remember to walk briskly to adequately stimulate the blood flow. Do your window shopping while cooling down.

Walking is usually an outdoor activitiy and in most cases determining the distance you walk is not difficult. Those who live in cities and suburbs can easily determine their mileage using a car's odometer or mileage indicator. Some of you will probably take advantage of a track; most outdoor tracks are 440 yards (a quarter of a mile) around. However, indoor tracks, (when available), will seldom be longer than an eighth of a mile. At times, distances may have to be estimated, especially if you use a shopping mall. But keeping track of the time you walk will give you some indication.

Regulating Your Walking Intensity

In the beginning of any exercise program it is important to take your pulse during and at the end of your workout session so you can regulate your intensity. After you have walked for as little as 10 minutes, stop and check your pulse. Also check your pulse at the end of the workout. It is important that you learn to find your pulse within a second or two after you stop walking. If you don't, your count will not accurately reflect your exercise heart rate. This may be difficult at first, but with a little practice it will become easy. (See Chapter 4 on how to take your pulse.)

It normally takes about ten minutes of walking before your heart rate levels out. This is the first time to check it. The key is to exercise near your target rate, not to exceed it. For most people (even if they have a low level of fitness) it is unlikely that a target heart rate of 75% of heart rate reserve can be reached as the result of walking. However, some people who walk at a good clip can reach 60% of their heart rate reserve. Combining this intensity level with lengthening the workout eventually to an hour provides a good stimulus for improving cardio-respiratory fitness.

Also check your pulse rate after you have cooled down for five to ten minutes. At this time your pulse should be near 100 or below. If not, it may indicate that you have worked too hard. Lack of sleep, illness, and climatic conditions (such as high humidity and temperature) can affect your heart rate not only during but after your workout. This is why it is important to monitor your heart rate so you can safely control your intensity level.

As you progress into your walking program it may not be necessary to check your pulse every day. With experience, you will be more attuned to the sensations of exercise and will be able to estimate your level of intensity without taking your pulse. During the early weeks, check your pulse regularly to see how you are doing and to make sure you are close to your target heart rate. For many, it is fun and intriguing to see how the heart responds to training. As you become better trained you will note a lower heart rate at the end of your walk. This is a good sign that you are ready to pick up your pace.

Avoiding Injuries

Most injuries that come from walking result from *overuse*. It's quite common to experience some aches and pains as you start out on an exercise program. Yet if you stick with our suggested sequence of walking workouts, these aches, if any, will last only a few days. If a pain persists in the toes or ankles, or in the joints of the knees, hips, or lower back, then there may be reason to be concerned. Often these pains relate directly to your shoes. Make sure you have good cushion and support. If you have flat feet, you may need some kind of arch support in your shoe.

Watch for sharp pains over the shin bone of the front of the lower leg (often referred to as *shin-splints*). There are many reasons for this condition. Frequently, they are caused by a weakness of the lower leg muscles. Quite often just putting a heel cushion or arch supports in your shoes will correct this. If this condition persists, you should see a specialist such as a sports podiatrist or an orthopedic doctor who is familiar with athletic injuries.

Also be on the alert for pains in the calf or thigh muscle. Often these result from overuse of the muscles (such as a pulled heel tendon). If these conditions clear up with continued modified walking, it was probably just a muscle injury. However, if you continue to have pains or cramping in the calves (only while you walk, not while you rest), then you may have poor leg circulation. This is cause for concern and warrants checking with a physician immediately.

The Walking Charts

The walking charts have three parts. Chart 1 is the *starter program,* which goes for 16 sessions, approximately four weeks. After completing this chart you should move to the *intermediate program* (chart 2) for an additional four weeks. After completing chart 2, you are ready for the *advanced program* (chart 3). The box on page 144 contains a summary of instructions for using the walking charts.

Remember, each session should be preceded by a warm-up of stretching exercises as described in Chapter 7. After you complete each vigorous walking segment, cool down with slow walking and some stretching exercises of the large leg muscles.

It is important to understand that the charts are just guidelines. They have been used for years and have worked for many people. Nevertheless, at times you may need to modify a day's workout, depending on how you feel. If you can't finish the prescribed work or walking distance for that day, then when you come back the next day or next session, repeat the previous day's workout until you can complete it.

On the other hand, some people adapt to the walking workouts more rapidly than others. I recall two women who began their training at walking chart 1, step 3. When they reached step 5, which calls for 32 minutes of vigorous walking, they were covering two miles in 30 minutes, which is a lot faster than the charts call for. Because of this favorable response to walking, I moved them up to the run-walk chart 1, step 1 (Chapter 9). This phase of the program is still predominantly walking, since it calls for 20 minutes of brisk walking before a series of four 35-to 45 second periods of running. I thought they could handle this, and they felt they were ready to begin some running. As long as you proceed with caution, you should feel free to modify the program to suit your progress.

It is a good practice to keep a record of your progress through the charts. As you complete each walking session, check the appropriate box on the chart and record your peak training heart rate. You may wish to also note your heart rate at the end of your walking session. Notations about the weather or how you feel are additional observations you may wish to jot down. Keeping an accurate record of your workouts can help you to stay with it.

The Starter Program

During the first four weeks we recommend four walking workouts a week; a Monday-Tuesday-Thursday-Friday pattern has been successful with us. Although you do not need to exercise every day, many of our walkers who are now on our maintenance program walk five to six days a week. However, I strongly recommend that at the outset you follow our four-day pattern. Rest days are important in all stages of training. Rest days allow your body to recover and adjust to the training stimulus.

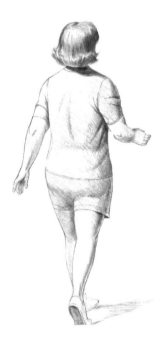

Missing one or more sessions because of illness or other conflicts calls for some adjustment when you resume your walking bouts. If you missed only a day or two, you may only need to drop back one session below the last one completed. If you have missed a week or more, then you need to make a greater adjustment. You may be tempted to disregard this advice. Don't! Failure to drop back may lead to unnecessary injuries and could endanger your health.

The purpose of completing the starter program is to enable you to walk two miles comfortably and to progress slowly to lessen the risk of injury to your previously inactive body. Once you have adjusted well to this task, you should strive to increase your distance, then to walk the distance faster.

The Intermediate Program

Once the starter program has been completed you will be walking continuously for about 45 minutes. This means you should be covering two miles or slightly more. In the intermediate program your goal is to walk three miles in an hour and then to quicken your pace so you can walk the distance in 52 minutes. Obviously your ability to walk three miles in an hour and then to walk it faster not only means a gain in fitness but a greater calorie output per minute of effort — a bonus for weight control.

The Advanced Program

When you reach the advanced stage of your walking program you will be covering three miles in 52 minutes (3.5 mph). It has taken you four to eight weeks, depending on where you started. If you desire to continue to walk (rather than beginning a walk-run program), the advanced walking charts provide you with two options. First, you can continue to pick up your pace and strive for the goal of walking three miles in 45 minutes (four mph) or you can increase your distance to four miles of walking in 70 minutes or less (approximately 3.5 mph). As you achieve these goals, your task is to maintain your walking program on a regular basis.

Varying your walking workouts from day to day is highly advisable. Finding new places to walk or varying the distances can help. For example, one day you might walk five miles or more, whereas the next day you could stride out on a three-mile walk at better than a 15-minute-mile pace. Innovations such as these will help diversify your walks. Keep in mind, your ability to walk four or more miles in an hour or less is a respectable accomplishment. Once accomplished, you may want to consider integrating some short running bouts into your workout. If you have been walking with the blessings of your doctor, you may want to check back with him or her first.

Is Running for You?

If you do not have any health problems, have not had any serious injuries from your walking program, and have had difficulty elevating your heart rate to the target level, then a gradual progression into a walk-run-walk program may be for you. In fact, if you are pleased with your improvement from walking, then no doubt you can also enjoy some running. Your walking workouts may have improved your fitness, but most likely you have not reached your physiological potential. The only way you can keep improving is to increase your exercise efforts. At this point, running is the most logical means to adequately do this.

Running chart 1 (Chapter 9) has been designed to introduce you gradually to running. At the start, short segments of running are inserted into your walking workouts. But if you don't want to integrate some short running segments into your regular workouts, then keep walking! To maintain your new level of fitness, you must continue on a regular basis (at least five times a week), keep up the intensity (reaching your target heart rate), and sustain each walking session for at least an hour.

USING THE WALKING CHARTS

1. *Warm-up with slow and easy walking* for three or four minutes, then do the stretching exercises. (Basic Twelve) to loosen and tone your main muscle groups. A cool-down period for five to six minutes is equally important.

2. *For your main conditioning session,* walk briskly for the designated time or distance listed in the charts.

3. *After ten minutes of walking, stop and check your pulse rate* for ten seconds and check it again at the end of your walk. Try to walk fast enough to keep your pulse rate elevated to or near your target rate.

4. *If you become winded, unusually tired, or your pulse rate is too rapid* (above your target rate) slow down to a more reasonable walking pace.

5. *The charts are arranged in steps.* A step represents two workouts (one workout per day), the second being a repeat of the first workout in the step. Providing you feel no adverse fatigue an hour after you have repeated the workout on the second day, you can move up to the next step. If your walking bout seems excessive, cut back to the previous step or continue repeating the workout you are on until you respond more favorably.

6. *The charts are designed so you will increase* your walking time four minutes (also your distance) every two days until you can walk for one hour (approximately three miles). Then you are encouraged to walk the same distance faster until you reach an advanced maintenance level.

7. *Once you have walked your way through the starter and intermediate charts,* you may be ready to include some short periods of running into your workout. If so, refer to the next chapter for additional instruction for making this change.

8. *Keep a record.* As you complete each workout session, check the appropriate box on the chart you are following. Also record your heart rate taken immediately at the end of your brisk walking. Keeping an accurate record of your workouts helps you to follow your progress from day to day systematically.

Chart #1
WALKING–Starter Program

STEP	SESSION	MAXIMAL MET CAPACITY	THE WORKOUT		DISTANCE GOALS (miles)	PEAK TRAINING HEART RATE	GENERAL COMMENTS
			VIGOROUS WALKING (min.)				
1	1 ☐ and 2 ☐	4 or below	15 to 20 min.		.5 to .8		
2	3 ☐ and 4 ☐		20		.9 to 1.0		
3	5 ☐ and 6 ☐	4.5	24		1.1 to 1.2		
4	7 ☐ and 8 ☐		28		1.3 to 1.4		
5	9 ☐ and 10 ☐	5.0	32		1.4 to 1.6		
6	11 ☐ and 12 ☐		36		1.7 to 1.8		
7	13 ☐ and 14 ☐	5.5	40		1.9 to 2.0		
8	15 ☐ and 16 ☐		44		2.1 to 2.2		

Chart #2
WALKING–Intermediate Program

| STEP | SESSION | MAXIMAL MET CAPACITY | THE WORKOUT | | PEAK TRAINING HEART RATE | GENERAL COMMENTS |
			VIGOROUS WALKING (min.)	DISTANCE GOALS (miles)		
9	17☐ and 18☐	6	48 min.	2.3 to 2.4		
10	19☐ and 20☐		52	2.5 to 2.6		
11	21☐ and 22☐		56	2.7 to 2.8		
12	23☐ and 24☐		60	2.9 to 3.0		
13	25☐ and 26☐	6.5	58	3.0		
14	27☐ and 28☐		56	3.0		
15	29☐ and 30☐		54	3.0		
16	31☐ and 32☐		52	3.0		

Chart #3-A
WALKING—Advanced Program
(Increase Pace)

| STEP | SESSION | MAXIMAL MET CAPACITY | THE WORKOUT | | PEAK TRAINING HEART RATE | GENERAL COMMENTS |
			VIGOROUS WALKING (min.)	DISTANCE GOALS (miles)		
17	33 ☐ and 34 ☐	7	50 min.	3.0		
18	35 ☐ and 36 ☐		48	3.0		
19	37 ☐ and 38 ☐	7.5	46	3.0		
20	39 ☐ and 40 ☐		44	3.0		

Chart #3-B
WALKING—Advanced Program
(Increase Distance)

STEP	SESSION	MAXIMAL MET CAPACITY	THE WORKOUT VIGOROUS WALKING (min.)	DISTANCE GOALS (miles)	PEAK TRAINING HEART RATE	GENERAL COMMENTS
17	33 ☐ and 34 ☐	7	56 min.	3.3 to 3.4		
18	35 ☐ and 36 ☐		60	3.5 to 3.6		
19	37 ☐ and 38 ☐	7.5	64	3.7 to 3.8		
20	39 ☐ and 40 ☐		68	3.9 to 4.0		

chapter nine

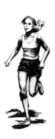

Running

A lot of people have a negative view of running. Some say that running is just a fad and is dangerous to your health. Such claims are misleading. On the other hand, the claims of spiritual rebirth and euphoric experiences by running enthusiasts are questionable. We believe that running, properly and carefully carried out, will yield beneficial results for you.

Many of the participants in our program at Ball State start with the walking charts because of their low level of fitness. After weeks of progressive workouts of brisk walking, they can handle a three-mile walk with ease. But for many of them, this improvement as the result of walking is not enough. They want to begin running because walking at a 15-minute pace or better is no longer providing an adequate training stimulus. At this point we introduce running into their workouts making it easier for them to train at their target heart rate (75% HR reserve). Eventually, they work up to running two to three miles, four or five times a week. This often happens to people who never thought it was possible even to walk for three miles when they started our program.

Selby waited until he was 68 before becoming active on a regular basis. His son and daughter-in-law were in our program and encouraged him to enroll. A physical examination revealed some abnormal electrocardiographic (ECG) changes. We had to begin at a low training level, so he began our walking program. He has progressively improved to where he now run-walks two to three miles each workout and feels great. Even though the ECG changes still occur during his physical tests, he has been able to improve his fitness capacity to a level well above other men his age. He is a good example of knowing your limitations and starting out properly.

Some people only walk for a couple of weeks before beginning to run. Others start running and walking right away. Where you start, of course, depends on your initial level of fitness. If you rate low in the initial tests, then your first workouts will involve more walking. Eventually you will be running more and walking less. Keep in mind the basic concept of alternating running and walking is to assure completing a certain amount of total work during the exercise session. Exercising at your target heart rate for a reasonable duration (30 minutes) is your goal.

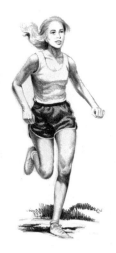

Fitness running isn't punishment! All the people running today wouldn't be doing it if it were unbearable. Agreed, many people *do* overdo it, and injuries, along with disillusionment, result. Much of the anti-running feeling results from the negative attitudes expressed about exercise that people remember from experiences in the past. I often hear people say, "I don't like to run because it's boring." Further questioning reveals that they never ran two days in succession in their lives or ran any further than a half-mile. Many are casualties from a crash program of running and expected miraculous results overnight.

Joann, a nurse, mother of four, wanted her husband, a physician, to join our program. He, in turn, suggested she join. She protested: "No, I could never do that." After further thinking and prodding from her husband, she decided, "Why not?" Joann, 48 at that time, recalled her first workouts: " I couldn't do one sit-up and I couldn't run more than 100 yards at a time." Now she does 20 sit-ups daily along with her stretching exercises and runs two miles, six days a week. She recalls with satisfaction running three miles with Patti Wilson during her run across the country for epilepsy. Not many 50-year-old women can make that claim.

Joann started out on a program similar to the charts in this chapter. She had some discomfort at first but nothing that hindered her progress. When recently interviewed she said, "Running just feels good. And, it's fun! I can do everything else better because I exercise. Years ago if you had asked me if I were active, I would have said yes. In retrospect, I didn't have any idea how *inactive* I really was. I always rode a bike but not far." Her advice to women (which is also appropriate for men): "You will be surprised how much more you can do than you ever thought you could do. I never dreamed I could run."

Some Preliminary Considerations

Up to now many of you have been following the walking program (previous chapter) and have progressed to where you can begin running. Because of your level of fitness (based on the tests in Chapter 5) some of you are starting out on your first workout. Presumably you are eager to begin running. However, some preliminary considerations are in order.

Selecting a Starting Point

The running charts presented in this chapter are based on over 20 years of actual experience with successful programs involving school children, college-age students, and adults of all ages. These charts make it easy for you to meet your individual needs regardless of your age, sex, or level of physical fitness.

Your beginning point on the charts is based on your maximal MET capacity. Those who have progressed through the walking charts and are ready to incorporate some running in the workout, can begin with running Chart 1 on page 166. Those who are just starting should be sure they can do the three-mile walk test in close to 45 minutes before starting a running program. If your fitness level is estimated at 7 METs or below, we strongly urge you to return to the previous chapter and begin a walking program at the designated spot on the walking charts. Many people see themselves capable of more exertion than walking. You may be! But let's not take any chances.

If your maximal MET capacity is 8 or higher, you can begin at one of the run-walk levels, as indicated in the table on page 166. Your first goal in a few weeks is to complete a run of ten minutes non-stop at your target heart rate. Eventually your goal will be to sustain a slow run of 20 to 30 minutes without stopping. Under normal circumstances this can be accomplished in 12 to 15 weeks of proper training.

Don't be offended at our suggestion that you begin with short, slow periods of running alternated with brisk walking. If you stay with the sequence on the charts, you will be pleasantly surprised how easy it is to improve and to progress without injury. Soon you will realize the good feeling and exuberance that comes from running, and you will be pleasantly surprised at how well your body adapts to each exercise step.

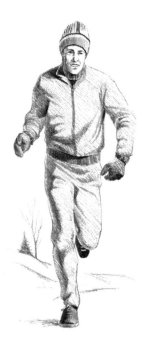

What To Wear

In his best-seller *The Complete Book of Running*, Jim Fixx covers from the ground up the basics on running gear and coping with varying weather conditions. I can especially identify with his observation that "some of the special pleasures (of running) come from being out in weather that drives more fainted hearted people indoors." Some of my most pleasant memories are of running during supposedly unfavorable weather — running through falling snow, running on a crisp, cold, clear morning as the sun rises, or running in a gentle rain. As Fixx states, ". . . there are few conditions under which it is impossible to run in comfort." Obviously your comfort depends on selecting the right running gear for different types of weather.

A usual tendency is to overdress in the winter cold. Your body generates much heat as you exercise, and you need less clothing than normal. It is important to keep your fingers and ears protected from frostbite. A good pair of mittens and a stocking cap will serve you well. Also a nylon or cotton/polyester windbreaker (with a full length zipper) is excellent as your outermost garment. Besides blocking the cold winds, you can take it off when it is not needed and tie it around your waist. I'm a believer that one of your layers should be a turtleneck jersey. As Fixx emphasizes, "always dress (for cold) so that your head and torso are warm."

I'm often asked whether you can freeze your lungs while running in cold weather. The answer is no. Research studies have shown that the air you breathe in is adequately warmed before reaching your windpipe and lungs. I have never heard of anyone injuring their lungs while exercising in cold weather. In heart patients, however, breathing cold air may cause chest pains. As a general rule, heart patients should avoid exercising in cold temperatures.

In warm weather it is best to dress with as little as you can get away with. Wearing white or light-colored clothing helps reflect the sunlight. By all means, don't wear rubberized jackets or pants to sweat off pounds. This only makes you lose water weight, not fat. Such clothing holds the heat in dangerously and can cause serious problems. A more detailed explanation concerning this matter is presented in Chapter 14. I hope you are not confronted with severe weather conditions (hot or cold, rain or snow) as you begin your program. Such conditions can be discouraging. As you begin to get in shape you will be better prepared to tolerate changing temperatures and weather conditions.

You do need proper shoes to run in. We have briefly discussed shoes in Chapter 6 and Chapter 8 (walking) so suffice it to say that running (or jogging shoes) are essential. Sneakers are too stiff in the forefoot, too low in the heel, and lack good side support for running. In Appendix B you will find detailed instructions for selecting and being properly fitted for walking or running shoes.

How To Run

The skill of running is often taken for granted. Frequently, the beginning runner starts plodding around a track or down the street without any instruction and wonders why it doesn't feel right. The repetitive cadence of an experienced runner looks simple and natural. But, the smooth and flowing interaction of the parts of the body while running represents an efficiency of movement for which there is no magic formula. However, certain practices can help you improve your running skill.

Proper posture while running is essential for good body mechanics. Good posture requires a good muscle tone. Regular adherance to muscle-toning exercises such as the Basic Twelve (see Chapter 7), as sit-ups, push-ups, and others (see Chapter 13), can lead to good posture and running mechanics. People with poor muscle tone and mechanics tend to let their belly sag, lean too far forward with their chest and head, and run with their buttocks projecting. Such a posture hampers a smooth and efficient running style. A good running posture entails an erect but relaxed body, head up, shoulders and hips level, with a relaxed arm swing and leg stride that allows the foot to fall directly under the body.

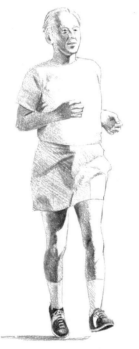 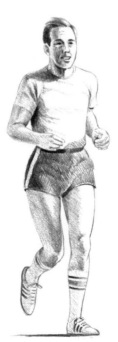 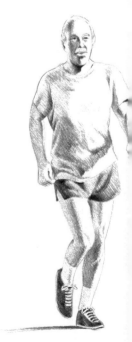

Over-striding is a common fault of many inexperienced runners. Over-striding results in the lead foot striking the ground ahead of the center of gravity, causing a jerky inefficient style. There is an optimal stride length for you. Finding it requires some experimenting on your part.

Other common faults are running with toes pointing inward or outward, excessive bouncing, carrying the arms and hands too high, and swinging the hands across the center line of the body. Strive to run as smoothly as possible, reducing all excess movements to a minimum.

Don't run on your toes. Many beginning runners start this way. Recently, a woman came to the lab complaining about acute soreness in her lower leg muscles and asked for help. Questioning revealed that a well-meaning friend had instructed her to run on her toes. This is not the way to run. The heel-to-the-ball or the flat-foot landing are the accepted ways for endurance-type running. These methods allow the maximum amount of shoe surface for landing. In both methods the foot should touch the ground as lightly as possible. In the flat-foot landing the entire outside of the sole meets the ground at one time. The heel (rearfoot) landing is quite similar except you set the outside of your heel down first, and roll your weight along the sole and push off with the ball of your foot. To say it another way, you run almost flat-footed, with your heel touching the ground slightly before the ball of your foot. A little practice will help you develop a smooth and efficient rhythm.

Running is a skill that can be improved just like any other athletic skill. Concentrate on maintaining an upright and relaxed posture, avoid overstriding, and don't run on your toes.

Where To Run

It's important to choose a good place (or places) to run. Stable and smooth surfaces are best since rough and uneven surfaces may keep you off balance and could lead to an injury. Try to choose a course that avoids heavy automobile traffic and its pollutants. If you have to run where there are cars and trucks, always run facing the oncoming traffic. If you run at night or in the early morning darkness, try to choose a course that has street lights. It's safest to wear bright-colored clothing and safety gear that reflects light.

It's helpful to explore a course by car (if possible) before you run it. Not only can you easily determine the mileage, but you may find obstacles, like hills or rough portions of a surface that you will be prepared for when running.

When you are away from home, it's best to ask others where to run. Unfamiliar territory may yield a number of surprises that can interfere with or interrupt your run. There are several interesting and informative books on where to run in most cities and towns in the U.S. as well as abroad.

Regulating Your Running Intensity

The key to a truly individualized running program is to find your own workload intensity or more specifically, your running pace. Throughout this book we have been recommending the use of your heart rate during exercise as a good index of exercise stress. On this premise, regulating your conditioning workload will depend on your heart rate response to the running sessions. Adjustments in the ensuing workouts, if needed, will be based on how you adapt to the training. The intensity of your running segments should be well within your capabilities, at approximately 75% HR reserve. After about five to six minutes of run-walks, you should determine your pulse rate within a few seconds of the end of the running segment. At the start, it is quite common for people to run too fast, causing the heart rate to rise above their target rate. Eventually you will be able to adjust your pace. Once you find your cruising speed, you will find it quite easy to stay well within your limits. For most people, the target heart rate is in the neighborhood of 140 to 170 beats per minute. At such a heart rate elevation, you should be able to carry on a conversation with a friend. If you cannot, you are probably exercising at too high a level of intensity. Slow down to a more comfortable pace.

Avoiding Injuries

Although running can be beneficial, it is high on the list of activities that cause injuries. Shin splints, knee pain, muscle pulls, tendonitis, and even fractures are quite common among runners. Fortunately, much more is known today about running-related injuries and ways to prevent them. It would be impractical to cover them all in this chapter. However, what follows are some common sense guidelines about avoiding running injuries.

Many running injuries are the result of overuse — doing too much, too soon. This is why I urge you to follow our recommendations for following the charts given later in this chapter. Your body needs time to adjust gradually to the exercise workloads we prescribe. You need to follow a systematic plan of increased workloads that your body can readily adjust to. It is common for enthusiastic devotees to ignore our suggestions and begin increasing the workout on their own. This extra lap or two can lead to injury. Our charts have been designed to lessen your chances of injury.

Expect some new soreness of muscles and joints during the first few weeks. These discomforts are the results of new demands on your muscles, even though some of you have been walking for as long as eight to ten weeks. Each activity you engage in involves a specific set of muscle groups. This initial discomfort, if you proceed properly, should not hinder your daily progress. Eventually this soreness will disappear. However, it may reappear as you speed up your program, add another exercise, or change to another sport or activity.

Always stretch before and after your workout. As you increase your capabilities to run longer and farther, you need to stretch more during your warm-up and cool-down. The Basic Twelve or similar stretching and toning exercises need to be a regular part of every workout. Although this is sound advice, many people (myself included) often cut down or even refrain from doing any stretching. However, having suffered from various running-related injuries over the years, I have recently become more faithful about warming up and cooling down. As a result, I have been able to reduce the incidence of injury.

Again, wearing proper running shoes is essential. This topic has been covered previously in Chapters 6 and 8. If you still have questions about footwear, I suggest you refer to Appendix B.

Avoid running on slanting surfaces such as sloping beaches or roadways. Continual running on such surfaces can cause stress on your leg muscles and feet. Streets are built with specific slants to allow water to drain off properly. Always running on one side means always stressing the body unevenly. If you can, switch sides periodically to avoid such stress. This means that at times you will be running with your back to traffic. Try to do this on less traveled streets and be careful.

Dr. George Sheehan, a cardiologist and running enthusiast, has always suggested that you should "listen to your body." I think this is excellent advise. However, our experiences in starting people indicate that most beginning runners are not able to recognize these signs at the outset. As you become better adjusted to working out, you will become more attuned to the workings of your body and will learn to distinguish between the discomforts of exercise stress and injury. Again, use your heart-rate response to your running sessions as a gauge of your intensity. Learn to anticipate and recognize signs of fatigue and exhaustion. Remember, rhythmic endurance-type exercise should lead to a state of mental and physical harmony, and each workout, although somewhat taxing, should *never* be torturing. Each workout, when completed, should leave you with feelings of accomplishment, relaxation, and a sense of renewed vigor.

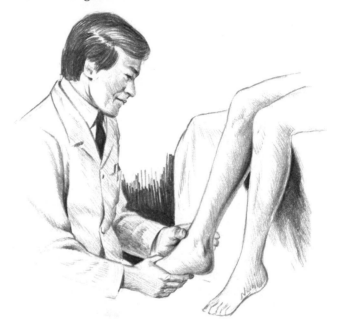

The key to avoiding getting seriously hurt is to recognize an injury in its early stages. Most sports medicine doctors categorize injuries as two basic types: acute and chronic. Acute injuries include muscle tears, fractures, and knee and ankle sprains. These injuries are usually caused by unexpected movements such as falling, turning quickly, or some sudden jolting action. Rest is usually the best remedy. Chronic injuries are more gradual and cumulative. Such injuries are difficult to recognize since they are not as painful at first. Often, people try to "run through" an injury, which is not wise. Usually if an injury persists or gets progressively worse, this indicates medical help is needed. Severe pain that lingers in a joint or bone needs professional attention. If you follow the charts and carefully note how you feel an hour or more after your workout, you can avoid most injury problems.

Even though you warm up and cool down faithfully and adhere closely to the charts, there is still a chance for injury. Many injuries arise from some imbalance of the body. For runners these imbalances do not show up until they begin extending their distances to beyond four miles. Fortunately, the science of sports podiatry has been able to effectively treat these imbalances of the lower extremities. Dr. Raymond Stidd, a sports podiatrist from Columbus, Indiana, has ably assisted our program in recent years. He is trained in the biomechanics of sports (the study of the mechanisms of movements). His approach, like that of an emerging group of podiatric specialists, is first to determine the causes of injury. If the cause is corrected, an injury is kept from recurring. Modifications of the shoe to correct an imbalance or a weak foot structure have helped many runners. Quite often, orthotics (shoe inserts made specially for your feet) are recommended. However, Dr. Stidd is quick to emphasize that, "orthotics are not the cure-all for everyone. Their purpose is to allow the feet to function in a more efficient manner." He recommends adherance to sensible training along with proper stretching and strengthening of the key running muscles. Specific exercises for off-setting the strength imbalances of the legs as the result of running are presented in Chapter 13.

Many books and articles are available today that are entirely devoted to running injuries. This is an indication of the concern for injury prevention. If you desire more detailed information about injuries and their prevention, I suggest you consult such sources.

The Running Charts

Running charts 1, 2, and 3 consist of systematically arranged workouts for assisting you to run continuously for 20 minutes within a period of 15 weeks. Chart 1 is the starter program, which goes for 20 sessions, or approximately five weeks. After warming up, your main workout consists of walking briskly for a designated time before beginning the run-walk segment of your workout. I must emphasize the importance of preceding your running segments with these brisk walks. We have found that this approach is very helpful in avoiding injuries during the early stages.

After completing step 10 of the first chart, you will be running (with brief rest periods) a total distance of about one mile. Chart 2, covering an additional five weeks, takes you to the point where your total running distance (again with abbreviated rests) will reach two miles. Now you are ready for chart 3, which brings you to the point where you can run *continuously* for 20 minutes, or approximately two miles. The box on page 164 contains a summary of instructions for using these charts. Each session should be preceded by a warm-up of stretching exercises as presented in Chapter 7. After you complete each workout, cool down with some slow walking and some stretching exercises of the large leg muscles.

Besides modifying your workout by lessening or increasing the running pace (intensity) you can also regulate workouts by varying the length of time of each run, the distance covered for each run, or the number of times you repeat your run-walk segments. There are ten steps in each chart, and each step calls for repeating the same workout the next session. Each run-walk workout is preceded by some walking followed by alternating short segments of running and brisk walking. When the run-walk segments are completed, a period of brisk walking is called for. As you advance through each step, the length of time of each running segment is increased, thereby increasing the distance you cover. Also, the number of sets of run-walks are planned so that each step requires a little more total work than the previous step. Some of the early steps in chart 1 are arranged so that you will do considerably more walking (up to as much as one mile) before beginning any run-walk sets.

The first three charts give no reference to distance. When beginning runners become preoccupied with distance, they are more apt to run too fast. As we have emphasized earlier, you want to go easy enough to conduct a conversation. Remember, our philosophy is to challenge your heart, lungs, and muscles vigorously, but well within your capabilities. Also, we want to spread your vigorous exercise over a period of 30 minutes or so. As you progress through the charts you will be sustaining your running longer. Eventually you will be able to run comfortably for 20 minutes non-stop. (See chart 3). In terms of distance, this will be anywhere from 1¾ to 2 miles, depending on your running speed. Now you are probably ready to think in terms of distance. Chart 4 helps you realize the goal of running continuously for three miles (or 30 minutes) at your target heart rate. This chart has worked well for many of our people. If you wish to strive for additional mileage, up to as much as six miles or more, you should progress slowly and not increase your total weekly mileage more than one or two miles. But first let's get you started properly.

When following charts 1, 2, or 3, it is important for you *to repeat each step for two days. If you recover fully and do not feel overly fatigued within an hour after the second day's workout, then move to the next step.* Reread the previous lines. These guidelines are very important to adhere to as you progress in your program. Be prepared to feel a little taxed as you near the end of your day's running workout. Each workout has been designed to require a gradual increase in effort as you progress through it. Under normal circumstances, you shouldn't have any trouble moving up a notch every two workouts. The basic idea is to gradually increase the amount of total running at each step, with less walking.

Be sure to walk briskly when the charts call for walking, even between your running segments. And don't overlook the importance of these walking segments between each run. A general rule: as your running distance increases, walk longer but do not walk for more than half the time of each preceding run. For example, if you run for two minutes, then your walking interval should not be longer than one minute.

If an overall body tiredness and fatigue lingers after you complete one of the prescribed workouts, this is a sign you are working too hard. Repeat the same workout until you recover more favorably. If you continue to be overly fatigued after your workouts, try running at a slower pace or move back a step. If this fatigue persists, then you should seek medical counsel. In most instances, if you closely follow these charts you will be surprised how easily you can do a little more every two days of workouts. Each step is designed to be more demanding and challenging as you progress from step to step. The intent is to exercise at a sufficient intensity to raise your heart rate to the target area. So run at your pace and learn to measure your pulse accurately. Remember, physical fitness is a lifetime pursuit, so start out slowly and progress gradually.

Before starting out you need to become familiar with the charts. At a glance, the charts may seem confusing. However, once you under-

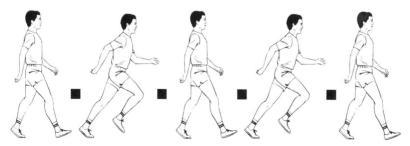

stand how to read them you will find them easy to follow. For example, refer to running chart 1, step 1. The workout begins with 20 minutes of brisk walking. Then under the "Run-Walk" heading you will notice it calls for running for 30 seconds, followed by a brisk walk of 30 seconds. This should be repeated four times (as indicated by the 4X). Then you walk for an additional ten minutes for a total exercise time of 34 minutes. Keep in mind this doesn't include the time for warm-up (The Basic Twelve) or the five minutes or so for a cooling down period of slow walking and some stretching.

Just to be sure you understand, skip down on chart 1 to step 9. This step calls for starting out with ten minutes of brisk walking followed by two runs of 45 seconds alternated with 30-second walks (2X). Then you do seven run-walks (7X) that involve runs of one minute duration alternated with walking periods of 30 seconds. At the completion of your run-walks you then walk briskly for six minutes, followed by your regular cool-down routine.

Once you have worked your way through chart 1, you will be running intermitttenly a distance of a little over one mile. Chart 2 is merely a continuation of this process in which the length of your runs is increased to time periods of two and three minutes. (See step 1). Your goal is to be able to do more running than walking and to prepare you to move into chart 3.

When you reach chart 3, you are getting close to the point where you will be able to sustain 10- and 20-minute running sessions. At this point you may wish to take a shorter walk than is recommended on the chart. For example, let's look at step 4, which calls for a three-minute run and a one-minute walk. You may want to walk for only 30 to 45 seconds between these running bouts. This is an individual variation that you might wish to do if you feel strong and ready for more running. As you look at chart 3, you will see that in steps 8 and 9 you are getting to the point where you can run a mile without stopping. For people in our program at Ball State, this has always been a very important day. When they reach this stage, they have a great sense of accomplishment.

Summary

It is important to understand that these charts are just guidelines. They represent a systematic approach for improving and enhancing your functional physical fitness. They offer you a simple approach to becoming a runner. These same charts have worked successfully for many people over the years, so stay with them and don't force it. They can work for you! Once you achieve your goal of running for 20 minutes (approximately two miles), you will fully realize it was worth all your efforts. At this stage you may wish to consider increasing your run to three miles or more. Chart 4 is provided for this purpose. A key point to keep in mind is be sure to continue running for 20 to 30 minutes on a regular basis in order to maintain a healthy and physically fit body. Remember, this is a lifetime program. It took much time and effort on your part to reach your goal. It will be much easier to maintain it.

Using The Running Charts

1. *Warm up with slow and easy walking* for three to four minutes, then do the stretching exercises (Basic Twelve) to loosen and tone your main muscles groups. Likewise, a cool-down period of walking and stretching is equally important for five to six minutes.

2. *For your main workout,* walk briskly for the designated time listed in the charts before undertaking the run-walk bouts. This part of your workout is very important in helping you avoid injuries that are common during early stages of most running programs.

3. *After you have completed a few of the run-walks,* check your pulse rate for ten seconds as you complete a run. Hopefully you will be near your target heart rate.

4. *If your pulse rate is too rapid (above your target rate)* slow down your running pace. Remember: you should be able to carry on a conversation as you run.

5. *The charts are arranged in steps.* A step represents two workouts, the second being a repeat of the first workout in the step.

6. *If your main workout of walking and run-walks* seems excessive, cut back on your running pace or move back a step until you respond more favorably.

7. *The charts are designed so you will systematically* increase your total work output every two days until you can sustain continuous running for 20 to 30 minutes. Then you are ready to consider runs of longer duration.

8. *Keep a record.* As you complete each workout session, make a check in the appropriate box on the chart you are following. Also record your heart rate taken at the end of your last vigorous running bout. Keeping an accurate record of your workouts helps you stay with it and enables you to systematically follow your progress from day to day.

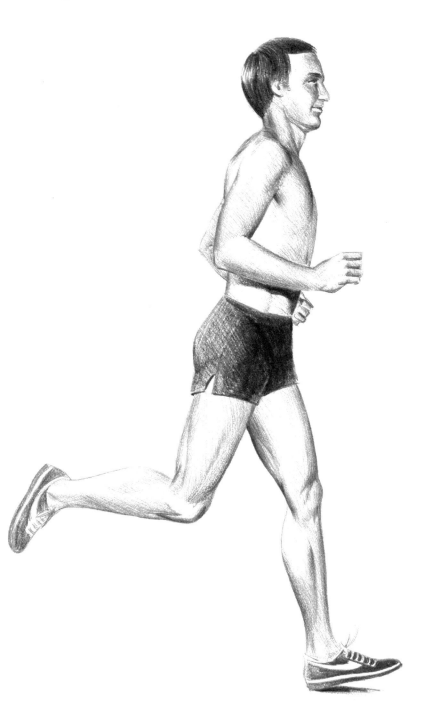

Chart #1 RUN–WALK

THE WORKOUT

STEP	SESSION	MAXIMAL MET CAPACITY	BRISK WALKING (min.)	RUN–WALKS	BRISK WALKING (min.)	TOTAL WORKOUT TIME (min.)	PEAK TRAINING HEART RATE	GENERAL COMMENTS
1	1☐ and 2☐	8	20	run 30 sec. and walk 30 sec. (4X)	10	33.5		
2	3☐ and 4☐		17.5	run 30 sec. and walk 30 sec. (6X)	10	33.0		
3	5☐ and 6☐		15	run 30 sec. and walk 30 sec. (6X) then run 45 sec. and walk 40 sec. (2X)	8	31.0		
4	7☐ and 8☐		15	run 45 sec. and walk 30 sec. (4X) then run 1 min. and walk 30 sec. (2X)	8	30.5		
5	9☐ and 10☐		12	run 45 sec. and walk 30 sec. (4X) then run 1 min. and walk 30 sec. (3X)	8	29.0		
6	11☐ and 12☐	8.5	12	run 45 sec. and walk 30 sec. (4X) then run 1 min. and walk 30 sec. (4X)	8	30.5		
7	13☐ and 14☐		10	run 45 sec. and walk 30 sec. (2X) then run 1 min. and walk 30 sec. (5X)	6	27.0		
8	15☐ and 16☐		10	run 45 sec. and walk 30 sec. (2X) then run 1 min. and walk 30 sec. (6X)	6	29.5		

Chart #1 RUN–WALK (cont'd)

THE WORKOUT

STEP	SESSION	MAXI- MAL MET CAPA- CITY	BRISK WALKING (min.)	RUN–WALKS	BRISK WALK- ING (min.)	TOTAL WORK- OUT TIME (min.)	PEAK TRAIN- ING HEART RATE	GENERAL COMMENTS
9	17☐ and 18☐	8.5	10	run 45 sec. and walk 30 sec. (2X) then run 1 min. and walk 30 sec. (7X)	6	30.0		
10	19☐ and 20☐		10	run 45 sec. and walk 30 sec. (2X) then run 1 min. and walk 30 sec. (8X)	6	31.5		

Chart #2 RUN-WALK

THE WORKOUT

STEP	SESSION	MAXI-MAL CAPA-CITY	BRISK WALK- (min.)	RUN-WALKS	BRISK WALK- (min.)	TOTAL WORK-OUT TIME (min.)	PEAK TRAIN-ING HEART RATE	GENERAL COMMENTS
1	1☐ and 2☐	9	10	run 1 minute. and walk 30 sec. (8X) then run 1.5 min. and walk 45 sec. (2X)	4	28		
2	3☐ and 4☐		10	run 1 min. and walk 30 sec. (6X) then run 1.5 min. and walk 45 sec. (4X)	4	28		
3	5☐ and 6☐		8	run 1 min. and walk 30 sec. (5X) then run 1.5 min. and walk 45 sec. (4X) run 2 min. (1X)	4	30		
4	7☐ and 8☐		8	run 1 min. and walk 30 sec. (2X) then run 1.5 min. and walk 45 sec. (6X) run 2 min. and walk 1 min. (2X)	4	32		
5	9☐ and 10☐		6	run 1 min. and walk 30 sec. (2X) then run 1.5 min. and walk 45 sec. (4X) run 2 min. and walk 1 min. (4X)	4	33		
6	11☐ and 12☐	9.5	6	run 1 min. and walk 30 sec. (2X) then run 1.5 min. and walk 45 sec. (2X) run 2 min. and walk 1 min. (6X)	4	33		

Chart #2 RUN-WALK (cont'd)

THE WORKOUT

STEP	SESSION	MAXI-MAL CAPA-CITY	BRISK WALK (min.)	RUN-WALKS	BRISK WALK (min.)	TOTAL WORK-OUT TIME (min.)	PEAK TRAIN-ING HEART RATE	GENERAL COMMENTS
7	13□ and 14□		4	run 1.5 min. and walk 30 sec. (2X) then run 2 min. and walk 45 sec. (8X)	232			
8	15□ and 16□		4	run 1.5 min. and walk 30 sec. (2X) then run 2 min. and walk 45 sec. (8X)	2	32		
9	17□ and 18□		2	run 2 min. and walk 30 sec. (8X) then run 3 min. and walk 1 min. (2X)	2	30		
10	19□ and 20□		2	run 2 min. and walk 30 sec. (6X) then run 3 min. and walk 1 min. (4X)	2	34		

Chart #3   RUN-WALK

STEP	SESSION	MAXIMAL MET CAPACITY	THE WORKOUT RUN–WALKS (Approximately 30 min. per workout)	TOTAL RUNNING TIME (min.)	PEAK TRAINING HEART RATE	GENERAL COMMENTS
1	1☐ and 2☐	10	run 2 min. walk 30 sec. (5X) run 3 min. walk 1 min. (5X)	25		
2	3☐ and 4☐		run 2 min. walk 30 sec. (3X) run 3 min. walk 1 min. (4X) run 4 min. walk 2 min. (2X)	26		
3	5☐ and 6☐		run 3 min. walk 1 min. (4X) run 4 min. walk 2 min. (3X)	24		
4	7☐ and 8☐		run 3 min. walk 1 min. (3X) run 4 min. walk 2 min. (4X)	25		
5	9☐ and 10☐		run 3 min. walk 1 min. (2X) run 4 min. walk 1.5 min. (2X) run 5 min. walk 2 min. (2X)	24		
6	11☐ and 12☐	11	run 4 min. walk 1.5 min. (2X) run 5 min. walk 2 min. (2X) run 6 min. (1X)	24		

Chart #3 RUN-WALK (cont'd)

STEP	SESSION	MAXIMAL MET CAPACITY	THE WORKOUT	TOTAL RUNNING TIME (min.)	PEAK TRAINING HEART RATE	GENERAL COMMENTS
			RUN-WALKS (Approximately 30 min. per workout)			
7	13☐ and 14☐	11	run 4 min. walk 1 min. (2X) run 8 min. walk 2.5 min. (2X)	24		
8	15☐ and 16☐		run 4 min. walk 1 min. (2X) run 10 min. walk 2.5 min. (1X) run 6 min. (1X)	24		
9	17☐ and 18☐		run 4 min. walk 1 min. (1X) run 10 min. walk 2 min. (2X)	24		
10	19☐ and 20☐		run 20 min.	20		

Chart #4 RUN–WALK

STEP	SESSION	MAXIMAL MET CAPACITY	THE WORKOUT RUN–WALKS	TOTAL DISTANCE RUN (miles)	PEAK TRAINING HEART RATE	GENERAL COMMENTS
FIRST WEEK 1	Mon. ☐		run 2 mile or for 20 to 24 min. walk 2–4 min. run .5 mile or for 5 to 6 min.	2.5		
2	Tue. ☐		run 1.5 mile or 15 to 18 min. walk 2 min. run 1.0 mile or 10 to 12 min.	2.5		
3	Thur. ☐		run 2.5 mile or 25 to 30 min.	2.5		
	F r i . ☐		run 1.5 mile or 15 to 18 min.	1.5		
SECOND WEEK 5	Mon. ☐		run 2.0 mile or for 20 to 24 min. walk 2–4 min. run .5 mile or for 5 to 6 min. walk 1 min. run .5 mile or for 5 to 6 min.	2.0		
6	Tue. ☐		run 1.5 mile or 15 to 18 min. walk 2–3 min. run 1.5 mile or 15 to 18 min.	3.0		

Chart #4 RUN–WALK (cont'd)

STEP	SESSION		MAXIMAL MET CAPACITY	THE WORKOUT RUN–WALKS	TOTAL DISTANCE RUN (miles)	PEAK TRAINING HEART RATE	GENERAL COMMENTS
7	Thur.	☐		run 3 mile or for 30 to 36 min.	3.0		
8	Fri.	☐		run 2.5 mile or for 25 to 30 min.	2.5		
9	Mon.	☐		run 2.5 mile or for 25 to 30 min. walk 2–4 min. run 1.0 mile or for 10 to 12 min.	3.5		
10	Tue.	☐		run 2.0 mile or 20 to 24 min. walk 2–3 min. run 1.5 mile or 15 to 18 min.	3.5		
11	Thur.	☐		run 3.5 mile or for 35 to 42 min.	3.5		
12	Fri.	☐		run 3 mile or for 30 to 36 min.	3.0		

T H I R D

W E E K

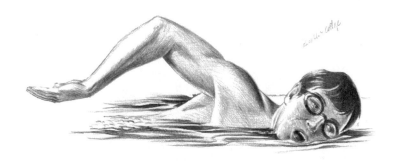

chapter ten

Swimming

Swimming is one of the best forms of physical exercise and an excellent alternative for people who can not or do not wish to run. Some people advocate swimming as the ideal conditioner because it contributes to total body development. Besides being an excellent means for developing cardiorespiratory fitness, it can be refreshing. The rhythmic movements of the muscles of the arms, legs and trunk and the stimulation of the cool water are highly beneficial to blood flow and muscle stimulation. The buoying effect of the water in a non-weight-bearing position spares the joints and muscles from wear and tear. Swimmers are less susceptible to the muscle soreness and tightness that are common to runners. Swimmers do not get the shin splints, tennis elbow, or torn ligaments that are common injuries with other sports activities. A simple variation of strokes permits not only an abbreviated rest to some specific muscles but allows other muscle groups to be actively exercised and stimulated.

Swimming does have its drawbacks. You must know how to swim! If you can't, we suggest you take advantage of the countless private clubs, YM/YWCAs, recreation centers, colleges, and public schools that offer instruction in swimming for people of all ages and abilities. The cost of qualified instruction in swimming is reasonable when compared with instructions in most other activities. Nevertheless, our experiences have shown that even if you are not a good swimmer at the start, you can still carry out a productive conditioning workout in the water. As you improve your skills, you can fully realize not only the conditioning benefits of endurance swimming but the pleasure and satisfaction of performing effectively in the water.

Another drawback to using swimming as a fitness mode is not having regular access to a pool. Being able to swim without interruptions in an open lane is a necessity. Fortunately more and more pool directors are setting aside certain hours during the day for lap-swimming. In Muncie, for example, the YMCA and our university have designated times for fitness swimming. In the summer the local outdoor pools are also providing lanes and specified times for lap-swimming. We are also discovering that this consideration for fitness swimming is becoming more and more prevalent across the country.

Patti, who has been swimming for five years, has progressed to where she can swim a mile a day during her lunch hour. This five-day-a-week, 29-year-old swimmer started out swimming just one lap at a time, with a rest period between the laps. Eventually she progressed to the point where she could swim a quarter of a mile before taking a rest period. After about four months she was able to cover a half mile without stopping. She leveled out at this distance for a couple of months until she felt comfortable. Then she worked on increasing her distance to ¾ of a mile, then to a mile. She feels that "when you begin a swimming program you have to have a lot of determination. At first I found it really hard and at times I wondered if it was worth the effort." She now says "I really enjoy the exercise and the swimming definitely helped me firm up my body. I find a swimming pool a place where I can meditate while working out. Actually I am able to work out a lot of my frustrations, and when I finish I feel better."

Now it takes her about 45 minutes to swim 1,800 yards, which is more than a mile. She varies her workouts at times by using a kickboard for one-third of the distance or at times backstroking a little to break up the routine of doing the freestyle, which is her predominant stroke.

There isn't an age limit to the enjoyment of swimming. For example, Will, who had a heart attack a few years ago, now swims a mile a day in about 40 minutes. This 61-year-old started about four years ago, and, as he puts it, "I don't dare stop." He has found swimming to be the best exercise to keep him fit and healthy. He says, "Swimming has helped me build up my endurance." Again, as we recommend to most people, he started out with repeat segments of swim-rests. Gradually the number of repeats are increased every two workouts. Eventually he worked up to where he could swim five or six laps and rest; then he reached his goals of a quarter mile, a half mile, finally a whole mile. "I enjoy swimming and I love the water," he says. "I feel so good after I swim because my body feels so relaxed." His philosophy is, "If you do young things and think young thoughts, you are going to last a little longer." Will is convinced that swimming for fitness is going to help him attain his desire of staying young.

Jim, a 38-year-old librarian at Ball State began our run-walk program a few years ago, but developed chronic soreness in his joints and knees that hindered his progress to the extent that he wanted to quit. However, he found his niche with the swimming program, and when retested after 12 weeks of lap swimming, he showed significant fitness improvements. He now swims anywhere from 40 to 50 lengths (1,000 to 1,200 yards) per session. Most important, he doesn't experience muscle or joint soreness any more. "I am now injury free," he says. "My muscles are more firm and toned up, and I have much more energy now than ever before. Some days I just don't feel like swimming, but after my workout, I feel refreshed and renewed for the rest of the day."

Swimming, when performed continuously and rhythmically, has great potential for developing and maintaining optimal cardiorespiratory fitness. The key to realizing a training effect still depends on your ability to work both at a suitable intensity and for a reasonable duration. To obtain maximum benefit from a swimming workout, you must develop a cadence (or a swimming pace) that challenges your heart rate, lungs, and muscles adequately. Just as in walking and running, your heart rate elevation as you swim is the key factor for regulating the intensity of your workout. Your cadence has to be substantially vigorous in order to elevate your heart rate to your 75% HR reserve level.

Swimming at a low level of intensity is quite easy. People who have good swimming skills and high body-fat (which makes them good floaters) can swim continuously without much effort. Unfortunately, they do not experience reasonable improvements in their physical fitness measurements. Swimming for these people can be compared to a leisurely bike ride through the neighborhood or a stroll through the mall. Their workouts are not sufficiently intense to produce a training effect. So keep in mind the importance of swimming at an intensity that is well within your capabilities but substantial enough to tax your physiological systems.

Some Preliminary Considerations

Some of you have decided to try fitness walking or running as a way to get in shape and are reading this chapter with the intent of using swimming as a way to mix your modes of activity. Or perhaps you have come to this chapter first because you prefer swimming as your fitness mode over walking or running. Others will choose this chapter because some physical ailment prohibits them from using walking or running as a fitness activity. Regardless of the reason, presumably you are eager to jump in the pool. However, some preliminary considerations are in order before you take the plunge.

Selecting a Starting Point

If you are just starting out and have recently taken an exercise tolerance test or our walking test, use your maximal MET capacity to determine your starting point by referring to the table on pages 78 and 79. For example, if you took our walking test and were not capable of walking a mile in 25 minutes or less, then you should start with swimming chart 1, step 1. If you are working your way through the walking or running charts and want to try swimming, note the chart and step you are presently on with that mode and then go to the corresponding chart and step in the swimming category. Given your progress with the other mode, you shouldn't have to start at the beginning with the swimming charts. However, if you're not a good swimmer or just beginning to learn, we suggest you start with chart 1, step 1. Because of your fitness condition with another mode, you may be able to progress more rapidly through the swimming charts. Just don't overdo it.

You will note that chart 1, step 1 calls for some brisk walking or running in water. Believe me, this can be quite vigorous. The water resistance makes movement through waist-deep water much more strenuous than moving at a similar speed outside the pool. Recent research at the University of Georgia indicates that substantial increases in breathing, blood flow, and energy needs are required when moving through the water at slow speeds. They found that approximately one-half to one-third the speed was required during walking and running in waist-deep water as compared to the same activity in air to elicit the same body responses. Also the researchers pointed out that the buoyant effect of water greatly reduces the weight-bearing stress on muscles and joints, an important factor for people with an arthritic condition or other joint problems. Walking in water is frequently used in the initial stages of cardiac rehabilitation programs. Also, it is an effective mode of exercise for those starting out with low levels of fitness.

What Equipment Do You Need?

Aside from a proper swim suit, you need only a pair of swimming goggles. They protect your eyes from the irritation caused by the chlorine and other chemicals commonly used in pools. Most sporting goods stores carry goggles. Be sure to find a pair that fits you and does not leak. Have an understanding with the proprietor that if they don't work, you can bring them back. About the only other wearing apparel you might require is a bathing cap. Again, select one that doesn't leak.

Additional accessory items might include a kickboard for kicking drills or small pulling tubes to wrap around your ankles causing a drag in the water for what competitive swimmers call *pulling drills*. Most pools have these accessories on hand.

How To Swim for Fitness

If you are not a very good swimmer, the distance from one end of the pool to the other may seem endless. If you are going to use swimming as a main part of your fitness training, it's wise to seek ways to refine your techniques. Even if you know how to swim, I suggest you enroll in a group class to brush up your skills and perhaps learn some new strokes to add variety to your workout. Dr. James E. Councilman, who has coached many Olympic and national champions, strongly feels that "efficient swimming seldom comes naturally." However, he feels that it's a skill that can be easily learned and fairly well mastered by anyone willing to devote a little time to it. It helps if you have someone who knows the proper mechanics of swimming to observe you and recommend ways to improve your skills.

The crawl stroke is the best stroke for fitness training. Nevertheless, to add variety to your workouts with segments of easier swimming, I suggest you learn the breaststroke, sidestroke, and some form of backstroke. It is not the intent of this chapter to provide swimming instruction, however, the following may help you recall some of the basics of swimming the crawl stroke.

Your body should be kept parallel to the surface of the water and in a streamlined position. Your head is partially submerged, with the water line just below your hairline. When you stroke, your body rolls on its long axis as if impaled on a spit. Doctor Councilman has observed in underwater motion studies that good swimmers roll at least 30° — some as much as 45° — off the vertical plane. However, too much rolling can slow you down. Also, the head should not be raised out of the water to breathe. Instead, the natural roll of the body on its long axis makes breathing easier on one side or the other. You should take in air (inhale) when your head is turned with the natural roll of the body. You exhale when your face is back in the water.

With the elbow slightly bent, the arm is angled into the water with the hand pulling the water downward and backward under the center line of the body. Each pull is completed with a pressing backward of the hand as the arm comes up alongside the hip. The kick is from the hips and thighs, not the knees. You should kick with short upward movements of the legs in a straight position. The feet act like flippers. Your major propulsion in freestyle swimming is derived from the arms, whereas the prime purpose of the leg kick is to stabilize the body in the water.

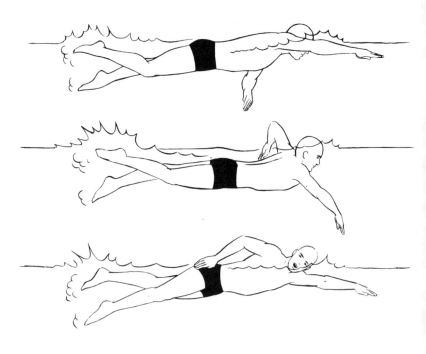

The crawl stroke.

Where To Swim

To swim for fitness, you need a pool or body of water that has lanes either marked on the bottom of the pool or roped off. Some of you may not realize just how easy it is to find a place to swim even in cold winter months. The most prevalent places are YM/YWCAs, but most fitness centers have heated pools and specific times for fitness training. The membership fee may be worth the convenience. If you live near a university or community college, we suggest you check on the availability of their pools. Often such an institution not only offers instruction to the public but also sets aside lanes for fitness swimming during off hours.

In choosing a place to swim make sure the facilities are well managed. It's best to have a certified life guard on duty during swimming sessions. If this is not possible, make sure that someone will be in the pool while you're there. Never swim alone.

In most pools the standard length of the distance from one end of the pool to the other is 25 yards. In this chapter a *lap* means the length of the pool, or 25 yards. If you use pools of shorter lengths, such as one in your backyard, you will need to modify the instructions in the charts of this chapter. For example, two lengths of a 40-foot pool is a little over 25 yards, so two laps in such a pool is one lap in our instructions.

Regulating Your Swimming Intensity

Swimming becomes a training exercise when it is done at a challenging intensity. Don't worry about how far you can swim continuously. Instead, be concerned with moving through the water at a speed that is vigorous enough to elevate your heart rate to your target level. Just as in walking, running, or cycling, the idea of training is to provide an adequate stimulus to your heart and circulation. Eventually your goal will be to swim continuously for 30 minutes or more. At first, think in terms of swimming one lap at a time. For example, in chart 2, step 1, we recommend that you first run in the water the width of the pool back and forth ten times, then swim one lap, then rest 15 to 30 seconds. Repeat this sequence four times. Once you can handle this task, go to the next step, which calls for adding two laps. When you can do 12 one-lappers alternated with periods of short rest, you are ready to start including some two-lappers in your workout (see chart 3). Don't worry about how fast you swim. Just be sure you find a rhythmical pace or speed that you can maintain reasonably well for the prescribed distance, whether it is one-lap or four.

Be sure to check your heart rate halfway through your workout and at the end. Many pools have a continuously running clock, often called a *pace* clock. It has a big second hand to help swimmers keep time of laps and rest periods and to check pulse rates. If you are nearsighted, you may need to have someone help you by calling out a ten-second time period for you. For example, as you stop at the end of the pool, immediately find your pulse. Your helper (with a watch or eyeing the clock) calls out "begin," and at the end of ten seconds, "stop." Now multiply this ten-second pulse rate by six to determine your pulse in beats per minute. For practical purposes the rate counted immediately following exercise is a good indication of your exercising rate in this particular stage of your workout. If your heart rate is above your target rate, swim your next segment less vigorously by slowing up. If it is below, then swim faster. Eventually you will begin to find out just how much effort it takes to provide a suitable stimulus to your heart. Then, you will be more able to perceive instinctively when you are swimming at your target heart rate, eliminating the need to check each day.

Depending on your swimming skills, age, and fitness status, it may take you several weeks or even months before you'll be able to swim for 30 to 40 minutes without stopping. However, by following the swimming charts you will soon be swimming more total laps, swimming more laps continuously, and getting stronger. You will be able to accomplish more and, just as in our experiences with walkers and runners, you will start to get excited about how your body has more energy and pep for everyday living. Remember our basic rule! Your workout should always be set so that you feel fully recovered and rested within an hour of its completion.

Swimnastics

Swimnastics is a term used to refer to activities and exercise performed while the body is submerged in water. The President's Council on Physical Fitness and Sports has coined the term *Aqua Dynamics* to describe such programs. Specific exercises and routines are carried out in the water for the purpose of enhancing muscular strength, endurance, and coordination. Although not as strenuous as lap-swimming, swimnastics is a means of exercise for individuals who are restricted because of painful joints or weak muscles. Exercising in the water is a common and viable form of training for the elderly and the physically handicapped. With less gravitational pull, along with the buoyancy of the water that supports the body and reduces its weight, movements are more comfortable and easily done. For the average person, significant improvements in cardiorespiratory fitness from a program involving *only* water exercises have yet to be demonstrated. However, for some people, it represents a starting point and for many, it can serve as an effective way to warm up before swimming laps. For persons who are more fit, such a program has merit as a supplemental program to lap-swimming.

As a general rule, many flexibility and calisthenic-type exercises, such as those presented in Chapter 7, can be modified so that a reasonable facsimile can be performed in the water. The following represents a sampling of some exercises that can be performed. Again, the vigor with which they are done and the number of repetitions performed will vary with the person. If you have a low level of fitness, a few weeks of doing these exercises along with some vigorous walking and running in the pool (chart 1) will be a logical starting point.

Fifteen swimnastic exercises are presented on the following pages. Whether you do warm-ups in the water or stretching exercises at poolside, they should always precede the more vigorous segment of your workout in the pool.

ARM CIRCLES

Much variation is possible here. Stand with feet apart, knees slightly bent so shoulders are just below water line. Extend arms to side, keeping them under the water. Use a variety of circular arm movements. Push and pull, forward and backward, downward and upward. Feel the resistance of the water.

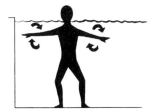

TRUNK TWISTER

Stand with feet apart, knees slightly bent
so shoulders are just below water line.
Twist trunk to the right with arms extended under the water then back to the left.
Rotate as far as you can stretch. Repeat
back and forth slowly with big sweeping
motions.

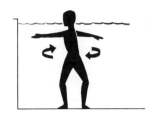

SIDE STRETCHER

Stand with feet apart. Bring one arm up,
overhead and toward the opposite side of
body. Slide other arm down the leg and
bending the trunk toward the lower hand.
Repeat back and forth with each arm.

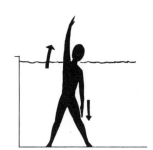

BACK STRETCHER

Standing, bend knee upwards, grasp
lower leg, and pull to chest. Hold for five
seconds. Alternate repeats with each leg.

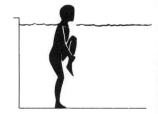

SIDE-LEG RAISES

Stand side to the wall, hold onto the edge
with near hand. Lift leg sidewards and
upwards from the hip. Pull down to starting position. Repeat ten or more times,
then turn other side to wall and repeat exercises with other leg.

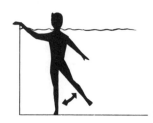

LEG-OVERS

Stand with back to the wall, reach back with arms extended and hold onto the edge. Lift one leg up and out away from the wall so that it is in front of body. Then rotate and cross the extended leg over the other leg as far as you can reach. Return leg to front extended position, then lower to starting position. Repeat back and forth alternating each leg.

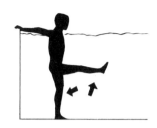

REAR LEG LIFT
(back extension)

Stand with hands on edge, chest to the wall. Pull leg back and up from the hip. Extend (point) the foot. Pull leg back. Alternate back and forth with each leg.

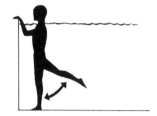

SCISSOR KICK

Float on your side, hang on with top hand holding gutter edge, bottom hand braced against the pool wall with feet below surface. Bring heels toward hips, bending at hips and knees into a crouched position. From this position spread the legs with the top leg extending forward and the bottom leg extending backward. When legs are extended and spread, squeeze them back together (scissoring). Pull with the top hand, and push with the bottom hand. The propulsive force of the kick will tend to cause your body to rise to the surface.

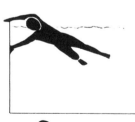

HEEL RAISES
(calf strengthener)

Stand facing wall and hold on for support. Bending at the toes, raise heels upwards and down. Repeat.

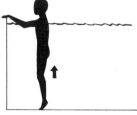

CALF STRETCHER

Stand facing the pool wall an arm's distance or less away with one leg forward
(knee bent) and the other leg back. With
your hands resting on the edge, bend your
elbows slowly allowing your body weight
to lean forward, back straight. Keep rear
leg straight, heel on bottom of pool so
that you will feel a stretching of the calf
muscles and heel tendons. Hold for five or
more seconds then bend the forward knee
even more, keeping heel on the bottom
and weight centered over the front foot
and hold stretch for five seconds or more.
Alternate weight back and forth a few
times and then repeat with rear leg forward, etc.

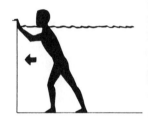

HAMSTRING STRETCHER

Facing the pool wall, raise one leg and
place your foot flat against the wall, keeping the leg straight. Reach and lean
toward the raised foot until you feel an
easy stretch on hamstring muscles (rear
thigh). Hold for five or more seconds.
Repeat a few times with each leg.

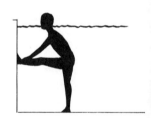

QUAD STRETCHER

Stand erect facing the pool wall, grasp the
edge with the right hand for balance. Lift
the right foot directly behind the body.
Hold the toes of the foot with the left
hand and pull the lifted leg up and back
until you feel a slight stretching discomfort in the upper front thigh (quadricep
muscles). Balance and hold firmly for five
or more seconds. Note, it is important to
stand erect, head up while holding the
stretch. Repeat a few times with each leg.

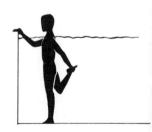

PUSH AWAY
(upper body and arm strengthener)

Stand facing pool wall at arm's length or more. Grasp edge with hands and bend arms so you are leaning toward the side of the pool. Push chest back by extending (straightening) your arms and pull body back to starting position.

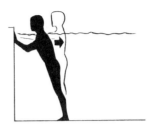

PULL-UP
(upper arm and body strengthener)

An effective way to improve upper body strength and endurance. You need to be able to grasp something solid that is at arms length above water level. (The handles on the diving blocks are ideal). Lower yourself in the water so that you are hanging from your gripping point. If your feet touch the bottom you will have to bend your knees and extend your feet backward in the water to avoid touching. Pull yourself up out of the water, and lower yourself back down. Repeat the exercise a few times.

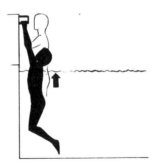

RUNNING

Try to submerge yourself so that you can move in a running gait with your arms and hands under the surface of the water. Walk or run as briskly as you can across the pool. The resistance of the water will help stimulate your heart and circulation.

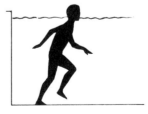

The Swimming Charts

We have provided six swimming charts. Charts 1 and 2 are starter programs, each involving 12 sessions covering approximately three weeks. You will note in chart 1 that there is no actual swimming involved; instead we have devised a program to get you accustomed to being in the water and exerting yourself. This chart is for people who have a low level of fitness or have limited swimming skills or both. This chart calls for walking back and forth across the width of the pool for a period of time. Then a series of running segments across the pool with short 30-second rests is introduced into the workout. Some may need longer rests than 30 seconds between each running segment. A variation is to follow each run across the pool with a walk in the water back across the pool during the rest period. Keep in mind that this is a beginning or a starter program. The purpose is to get you used to exercising in water.

Chart 2 starts you out running some widths of the pool followed by swimming lengths of the pool. Note in the chart the suggestions to swim a lap and rest for 15 to 30 seconds, then swim back the length of the pool. As mentioned earlier a length is referred to as a lap and in most pools this is equivalent to 25 yards. Also in chart 2 you will notice after every two sessions you will be increasing the total distance swum by 50 yards. Eventually (step 6) you will be able to swim a total distance of 300 yards.

Chart 3 does not involve any running in the water, and for many people this may be the most reasonable starting point. In general, you will alternate swimming laps with short rest periods. Eventually you will be swimming some two-lappers without stopping. At the end of 12 sessions (another three weeks) you will be swimming approximately 600 yards. As in chart 2 you will be increasing your total swimming distance 50 yards every two workouts, or an additional 100 yards per week. Charts 4 and 5 follow a similar pattern. Gradually, you will keep getting stronger each day and over a period of 12 to 15 weeks you will be putting in a substantial workout each day. Chart 6 continues chart 5 to where you are swimming close to a mile in total distance, or four laps (100 yards) at a time, followed by brief rests. Of course, if at this stage you can swim without rests, keep going.

Remember, each session should be preceded by a warm-up of stretching exercises either on the pool deck using the Basic Twelve or in the water using the swimnastic exercises presented in this chapter. Be sure to cool down with easy swimming and slow stroking after each workout. Walking on the pool deck together with some stretching exercises of the major muscle groups of the body is another possibility for cooling down.

It is important that you understand that the charts are just guidelines. We have used them in advising people who have chosen swimming as their fitness mode. If you can't finish the prescribed swimming bout each day, then you should repeat the workout at your next session until you can complete it.

One difficulty in prescribing swimming workouts for people is the wide differences in swimming skill. Those who possess good swimming skill often move through the charts more rapidly than others. As long as you proceed with caution, you should feel free to modify your program to suit your capabilities. However, we suggest you keep a record of your progress through the charts. As you complete each swimming session, check the appropriate box on the chart and record your training heart rate. Keeping an accurate record of your workouts will not only help you stay with it, but keep you from doing too much, too soon. Systematic training with gradual increases will assure reasonable gains in endurance without unnecessary fatigue.

When you miss one or more sessions because of illness or other conflicts you need to make some adjustment when you resume your swimming exercise. If you missed only a day or two you may only have to drop back one session or repeat your most recent session. If you miss a week or more, then you need a greater adjustment. You may be tempted to disregard this advise. Don't! Failure to drop back or make adjustments when you have missed some of your regular swimming sessions can lead to unnecessary fatigue, stress, and possible injury. Remember, the key is to gradually increase the amount of swimming that you do each day.

Using The Swimming Charts

1. *Start out by warming up* with some of the swimnastic stretching exercises in water at chest or waist depth. Use this period for getting your body adjusted to the water along with loosening and activating your main muscle groups. Also, when your main conditioning segment is complete, repeat some of these exercises during your cool-down.

2. *The swimming charts provide* a systematic pattern of steps designed so you will increase your swimming time and distance in a graduated manner every two days.

3. *The charts are arranged in steps.* A step represents two workouts, the second being a repeat of the first workout in the step.

4. *Providing you feel no adverse fatigue* one hour after you have repeated the workout on the second day, you can move up to the next step. If your swimming segments seem excessive, cut back to the previous step or continue repeating the step you are on until you respond more favorably.

5. *If you are starting out with chart 1* (walking and running in the water) your workouts will be most effective if you submerge your body so the arms and elbows are kept under water. Walk and run at a pace that is taxing and also sufficient to elevate your pulse rate to near your target level.

6. *If during the suggested time period of rest,* you do not recover reasonably well, take a longer rest before swimming your next segment.

7. *At the end of each chart you are encouraged* to swim the designated distance as continuously as possible with rest periods when you wish. (See session 11 and 12 on each chart).

8. *Once you have swum your way through the charts,* you are ready to extend your workouts to include more continuous swimming. Your ultimate goal is to be able to swim continuously (without a rest period) a half-mile (880 yards) or more.

9. *Keep a record.* As you complete each workout session, check the appropriate box on the chart you are following. Also record your heart rate taken at the end of your last vigorous swimming lap. Keeping an accurate record of your workouts helps you stay with it and enables you to systematically follow your progress from day to day.

Chart #1 SWIMMING
WALKING AND RUNNING IN WATER

THE WORKOUT

STEP	SESSION	WALK (widths)	RUN–REST (widths)	WALK (widths)	TOTAL WORK-OUT TIME (min.)	TRAIN-ING HEART RATE	GENERAL COMMENTS
1	1 ☐ and 2 ☐		Run across the pool, rest 30 sec. (6X)	10 min.	24 to 30		
2	3 ☐ and 4 ☐	8 min.	Run across the pool, rest 30 sec. (6X)	10 min.	24 to 30		
3	5 ☐ and 6 ☐	6 min.	Run across the pool, rest 30 sec. (8X)	10 min.	24 to 30		
4	7 ☐ and 8 ☐	4 min.	Run across the pool, rest 30 sec. (10X)	10 min.	24 to 30		
5	9 ☐ and 10 ☐	2 min.	Run across the pool, rest 30 sec. (12X)	10 min.	24 to 30		
6	11 ☐ and 12 ☐		Run back and forth a total of 15 widths, rest when needed but no longer than 20 to 30 sec.				

Chart #2 SWIMMING
RUNNING AND SWIMMING

THE WORKOUT

STEP	SESSION	RUN (widths)	SWIM-REST (lengths)	WALK (widths)	TOTAL WORK-OUT TIME (min.)	APPROXI-MATE TOTAL DISTANCE SWAM (yd.)	TRAIN-ING HEART RATE	GENERAL COMMENTS
1	1☐ and 2☐	10X with rest when needed	Swim 1 lap, rest 15 to 30 sec. (4X)	6 min.	20-30	100		
2	3☐ and 4☐	8X with rest when needed	Swim 1 lap, rest 15 to 30 sec. (6X)	5 min.	20-30	150		
3	5☐ and 6☐	6X with rest when needed	Swim 1 lap, rest 15 to 30 sec. (8X)	4 min.	20-30	200		

Chart #2 SWIMMING
RUNNING AND SWIMMING (cont'd)

4	7☐ and 8☐	4X with rest when needed	Swim 1 lap, rest 15 to 30 sec. (10X)	3 min.	20-30	250	
5	9☐ and 10☐	2X with rest when needed	Swim 1 lap, rest 15 to 30 sec. (12X)	2 min.	20-30	300	
6	11☐ and 12☐	2X with rest when needed	Swim a total of 12 laps rest when needed but no longer than 15 to 30 sec.		20-30	300	

Chart #3 SWIMMING
SWIM-REST

THE WORKOUT

STEP	SESSION	SWIM-REST	TOTAL WORK-OUT TIME (min.)	APPROXI-MATE TOTAL DISTANCE SWAM (yd.)	TRAIN-ING HEART RATE	GENERAL COMMENTS
1	1☐ and 2☐	Swim 1 lap, rest 15 to 30 sec. (10X) Swim 2 laps, rest 45 sec. (2X)	24 to 28	350		
2	3☐ and 4☐	Swim 1 lap, rest 15 to 30 sec. (8X) Swim 2 laps, rest 45 sec. (4X)	24 to 28	400		
3	5☐ and 6☐	Swim 1 lap, rest 15 to 30 sec. (6X) Swim 2 laps, rest 45 sec. (6X)	24 to 30	450		
4	7☐ and 8☐	Swim 1 lap, rest 15 to 20 sec. (4X) Swim 2 laps, rest 45 sec. (8X)	24 to 30	500		
5	9☐ and 10☐	Swim 1 lap, rest 15 sec. (2X) Swim 2 laps, rest 30 to 45 sec.	24 to 30	550		
6	11☐ and 12☐	Swim a total of 24 laps, resting when needed but no longer than 15 to 30 sec.	24 to 35	600		

Chart #4 SWIMMING
SWIM-REST

STEP	SESSION	THE WORKOUT — SWIM–REST	TOTAL WORKOUT TIME (min.)	APPROXIMATE TOTAL DISTANCE SWAM (yd.)	TRAINING HEART RATE	GENERAL COMMENTS
1	1 ☐ and 2 ☐	Swim 2 laps, rest 20 to 30 sec. (10X) Swim 3 laps, rest 30 sec. (2X)	22 to 30	650		
2	3 ☐ and 4 ☐	Swim 2 laps, rest 20 sec. (8X) Swim 3 laps, rest 30 sec. (4X)	24 to 32	700		
3	5 ☐ and 6 ☐	Swim 2 laps, rest 20 sec. (6X) Swim 3 laps, rest 30 sec. (6X)	26 to 36	750		
4	7 ☐ and 8 ☐	Swim 2 laps, rest 10 sec. (4X) Swim 3 laps, rest 20 to 30 sec. (8X)	28 to 36	800		
5	9 ☐ and 10 ☐	Swim 2 laps, rest 10 sec. (2X) Swim 3 laps, rest 20 to 30 sec. (10X)	30 to 38	850		
6	11 ☐ and 12 ☐	Swim a total of 34 laps, rest when needed but no longer than 20 to 30 sec.	24 to 40	850		

Chart #5 SWIMMING
SWIM–REST

STEP	SESSION	THE WORKOUT SWIM–REST	TOTAL WORKOUT TIME (min.)	APPROXIMATE TOTAL DISTANCE SWAM (yd.)	TRAINING HEART RATE	GENERAL COMMENTS
1	1 ☐ and 2 ☐	Swim 3 laps, rest 20 sec. (9X) Swim 4 laps, rest 30 sec. (2X)	28 to 34	825		
2	3 ☐ and 4 ☐	Swim 3 laps, rest 20 sec. (8X) Swim 4 laps, rest 30 sec. (3X)	28 to 34	950		
3	5 ☐ and 6 ☐	Swim 3 laps, rest 20 sec. (7X) Swim 4 laps, rest 30 sec. (4X)	28 to 35	925		
4	7 ☐ and 8 ☐	Swim 3 laps, rest 10 sec. (6X) Swim 4 laps, rest 20 to 30 sec. (5X)	28 to 35	950		
5	9 ☐ and 10 ☐	Swim 3 laps, rest 10 sec. (5X) Swim 4 laps, rest 20 to 30 sec. (6X)	28 to 36	975		
6	11 ☐ and 12 ☐	Swim a total of 40 laps, rest when needed but no longer than 20 to 30 sec.	30 to 40	1000		

Chart #6 SWIMMING
SWIM–REST

STEP	SESSION	THE WORKOUT SWIM–REST	TOTAL WORKOUT TIME (min.)	APPROXIMATE TOTAL DISTANCE SWAM (yd.)	TRAINING HEART RATE	GENERAL COMMENTS
1	1 ☐ and 2 ☐	Swim 4 laps, rest 20 to 30 sec. (6X) Swim 6 laps, rest 30 sec. (3X)	30 to 38	1050		
2	3 ☐ and 4 ☐	Swim 4 laps, rest 20 sec. (5X) Swim 6 laps, rest 30 sec. (4X)	30 to 38	1100		
3	5 ☐ and 6 ☐	Swim 4 laps, rest 20 sec. (4X) Swim 6 laps, rest 20 to 30 sec. (5X)	32 to 40	1250		
4	7 ☐ and 8 ☐	Swim 4 laps, rest 10 sec. (3X) Swim 6 laps, rest 20 sec. (6X)	34 to 42	1400		
5	9 ☐ and 10 ☐	Swim 4 laps, rest 10 sec. (2X) Swim 6 laps, rest 10 to 20 sec. (7X)	36 to 44	1550		
6	11 ☐ and 12 ☐	Swim a total of 64 laps, rest when needed but no longer than 20 to 30 sec.	40 to 48	1600		

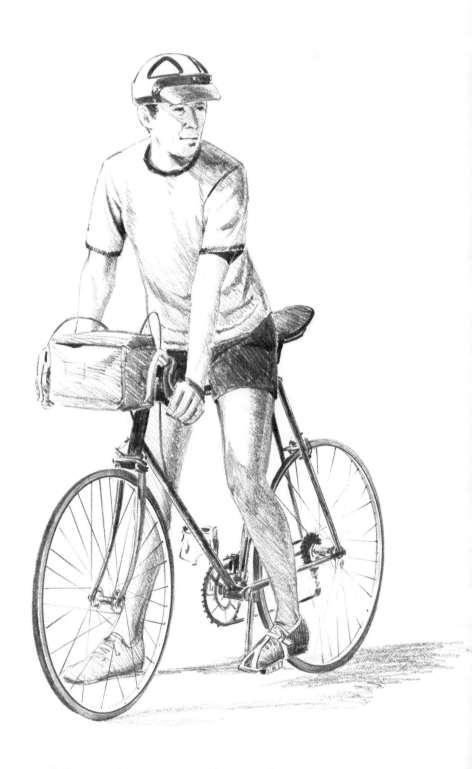

chapter eleven

Bicycling

Do you recall when you first learned how to ride a bike? In my childhood we didn't have training wheels, so after struggling for days on my friend's bike, I decided to get on and pedal as fast as I could, hoping the speed would keep me up. It worked! The joy of that accomplishment I well remember today. In fact, I can recall the spontaneity and the fun of hopping on my bike to get from here to there. It was simply the natural thing to do. But I retired my one speed when I became a teenager because it just wasn't "cool" to ride a bike then.

Times have changed. Many of us have rediscovered the bicycle. There's never been a better time to own and ride a bicycle. With higher gas prices, increased traffic jams, and higher auto repair bills, a bicycle provides a practical alternative to the automobile. Not only is using a bicycle healthy for out pocketbooks and environment, it also does not pollute the air.

A bicycle can be used for transportation, touring, racing, and physical fitness training, as well as for recreation. A bike is a weekend plaything for some, but for others it provides daily transportation. And many are using it as an alternative to running because the cardiorespiratory benefits of cycling can equal the benefits of running.

For sure, bicycling for physical fitness requires more exertion than is needed in everyday situations like pedaling to the grocery for a loaf of bread. Leisurely pedaling will not benefit your fitness. However, vigorous, sustained pedaling (but well within your abilities) can stimulate your lungs, heart, and muscles adequately for fitness gains. Racing requires an even higher level of physical fitness, and many hours of riding (conditioning) are necessary if you want to be competitive. Most of us do not want to race, but touring and vigorous pleasure riding can do much for developing and maintaining physical fitness. Naturally, the speed at which you ride, just as in walking and running, will govern the fitness benefits of cycling. In general, riding at a pace of four to five minutes a mile (12 to 15 mph), equivalent to a 75% HR reserve intensity for most people for a good 30- to 60- minute workout is a reasonable goal and will provide an adequate training stimulus for the cardiorespiratory system.

Enthusiasm for bicycle touring is booming. One touring entrepreneur calls the bicycle the RV (recreation vehicle) for the '80s. More and more people are finding bicycle tours not only pleasurable but a way to experience the countryside as motorized travelers never do. Most mapped bike routes are on rural roads that take you through the heart of small towns. You can choose to rough it by camping and cooking in the outdoors or spend your evenings at comfortable accommodations with prepared meals. Usually, tours are organized with enough route options so you can decide for yourself how strenuous you want the day's trip to be. But first you must get in shape so you can enjoy the many possibilities for expanding your world on a bicycle.

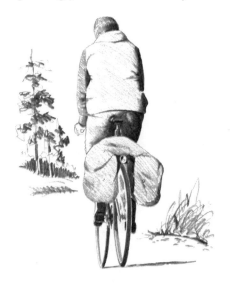

Some Preliminary Considerations

Selecting a Starting Point

The ultimate aim of a cycling fitness program is to train your body so you can steadily pump your legs at a rate sufficient to adequately challenge your cardiorespiratory system for 30 to 60 minutes. As a general rule, your first few weeks of training should consist of a moderate riding pace so your leg muscles and overall body functions can adjust reasonably well to these new stresses. Even if you have progressed well in other fitness modes and want to try cycling as an alternative, you should start with moderate training. Walking, running, or swimming will not adequately prepare your leg and thigh muscles for the rigors of fitness cycling. As with other fitness modes, you should try to avoid unnecessary injuries that result from doing too much, too soon.

As we recommend for the walking, running and swimming programs, before you start your cycling program, you need an accurate assessment of your physical condition. This means a medical or fitness checkup by a doctor with knowledge of sports medicine, as suggested in Chapter 5. A checkup at a fitness center with qualified personal (MD and exercise physiologist) will provide you with the best assessment. If this is not possible, our walking test (See Chapter 5) will help you select a starting point in our cycling charts. If you have not been active in recent months, your first few weeks of riding will be at relatively low to moderate speeds with a gradual build-up of total distance each session. You want to reach the point where you will be able to sustain a continuous ride for 30 minutes. Such an effort, we feel, is comparable to walking briskly for an hour. Once this is accomplished, you are ready to begin a more vigorous training regimen (see chart 1) aimed at helping you reach your fitness potential.

What To Wear

Improper clothing can be a hindrance as well as a source of discomfort during your cycling workout. For the serious cyclist, street clothes are improper and too confining for efficient and enjoyable cycling. Clothing specifically designed to maximize comfort and mobility is more practical and pleasurable. Of course, you don't need a special outfit to begin a bicycling fitness program, but as you get into it, you will discover that cycling in regular shoes and clothing will not do. For example, you will soon realize that tight-fitting jeans hinder movement. Well-designed cycling clothes have various features to make them most suitable for the sport. In general, bicycle wear should be light-weight, streamlined, unrestricting, protective, and durable. Of course, the items you need depend on how far you travel, how often, the climatic conditions, your level of participation (beginner, tourer, racer) and of course, your budget.

Some items you should consider buying first are cycling shorts, jerseys, shoes, and headgear. Toe clips and straps and cycling gloves are other items that become more important as you become more serious about cycling. Bicycle wear comes in varying types of fabrics made of natural fibers (wool and cotton), synthetic fibers (acrylic, polyesters, and nylon), and blends. Your personal needs and preferences regarding design, weight, elasticity, permeability, and absorption will effect your decision on what to buy.

Let's look at what makes good cycling shorts and jerseys. The legs on the shorts should be long enough to keep the skin on your legs from rubbing against the saddle. The body of the shorts should be a blend of wool and polyester (or polyester and acrylic). Seams should be flat to avoid abrasion. Sewn into the seat area of your shorts should be a large, thick, and fluffy chamois. This provides a soft cushiony area between you and the saddle. Some shorts come with a terry cloth crotch liner to prevent chafing. Most cycling jerseys are cut long to keep your back covered as you lean forward in a riding position.

According to avid participants, cycling shoes are a sadly underutilized accessory. Many people use running shoes. However, the cyclists say you have to try the specially made cycling shoe with its stiff shank to realize how much better your feet will feel. Manufacturers are now beginning to design shoes for the touring cyclist and physical fitness advocate. At this point, some are making a good no-frills cycling shoe without expensive leather or manufacturing techniques. Basically, one popular brand is an all-canvas refinement of the racing shoe but without a steel shank in the sole. It has a stiff sole (a contrast from the running shoe which should be very flexible) in order to spread the pedaling pressure around the whole foot rather than allowing the pressure to concentrate in one spot. The canvas upper part of this shoe is reinforced with rubber. The rubber sole (a cleatless cleat) does not slip and helps to maintain good contact with the pedals. Another brand of touring shoes is nylon reinforced with leather. Obviously, well-fitting socks are critical. A sloppy fit or a too tight fit can lead to blisters and other foot problems. Ventilation holes and adequate padding where the toestrap passes over the foot are important considerations when you buy cycling footwear.

Although not needed for the beginning cyclist, toe clips (with toe straps) will make you a more efficient rider. The toe clip is a strong, spring-steel fixture that is bolted to the front side of each pedal with a leather top strap and buckle. It is designed to provide a fixed position for the foot. When your feet are attached to the pedals, you can push down with one leg while pulling up with the other. Until you become accustomed to the toe clips and straps, you should not tighten the straps. At first, you may find it difficult to get your feet in and out of the toe clips when you suddenly have to stop. Obviously this could cause a potentially dangerous fall. However, once you learn to tighten and loosen the toe straps while riding, the danger of falling when stopping will be eliminated.

Avid cyclists feel that riding without a helmet is ridiculous. Many cyclists who have fallen have been saved from serious injury because they wore protective headgear. The best-made helmets are lightweight and well-ventilated with excellent shock-absorbing qualities and a sturdy chin strap. It should permit the wearer to hear well. Also, cycling gloves with added padding are essential and a great protection in a crash or fall. Of course riding in the cold, heat, or rain requires additional considerations for cycling wear.

Selecting a Bike

The question is often asked, "Do I need a ten-speed, with that skinny saddle, upside-down handle bars, and a complicated gear system to attain fitness?" Years ago my reaction to that question was an emphatic no! My cycling friends were somewhat critical of my lack of acceptance of the jazzier ten-speeds. However, with encouragement from my teenage daughter, I weakened and bought one. I must admit I have found it to be a very functional and efficient piece of equipment. You don't need a ten-speed to attain fitness, but if you become a serious cyclist, you'll find it more practical than the single-speed or three-speed bike.

You do need a bike in good mechanical condition. More than a million people are injured in bicycle accidents each year, and roughly 1,000 of them die. Many of these accidents are caused by faulty equipment (and poor cycling techniques). The U.S. Consumer Product Safety Commission, in order to reduce the number of bicycle accidents, has set rigid safety standards for all bicycles marketed today. Therefore, your bike should be in good working condition and meet the commission's standards.

The success of your cycling fitness program requires not only a good bicycle but one adjusted properly for your body. Getting the full fitness benefits from cycling depends largely on the position of your body on the bike. Saddle height, handlebar height, frame size, and stem length are important. An improperly fitted bike can cause all sorts of muscle and joint strains, and keep you from developing sound bike-handling skills.

If you plan to buy a new bike, go to a shop that specializes in bicycles; not one that just sells them, but one that repairs them as well. You can buy a bike at a department store and probably save money. But by making your purchase at a bike specialty shop, you can expect to have the bike adjusted to your body size and reasonable repair and maintenance service. The bike shop proprietors are well trained in fitting you properly to your bike and keeping the bike in good condition.

Don't let the sophisticated chain wheel and the sprocket arrangement on the ten-speed scare you away. All you need to know is that there are two gear-shift levers: one controlling the chain wheel in the front, which has two sprockets; and one controlling the free wheel in the rear, which has five sprockets. By moving the levers up and back while you pedal, you engage any one of ten gears. These gear-shift levers are operating what is called a *derailleur* system. The derailleur is the part that shifts gears. In other words it derails the chain from one sprocket to the next. In most systems, pushing the left lever away from you and pulling the right lever toward you will put your bike into a lower (easier to pedal) gear. After a few minutes of riding and practicing, you will become familiar with which way to move the levers for easier pedaling and which way to move them for harder pedaling. As you operate the levers you may hear the chain rattling. This can be quite annoying and is an indication that you are not in gear. By moving the lever forward or back a little, the chain will properly seat itself.

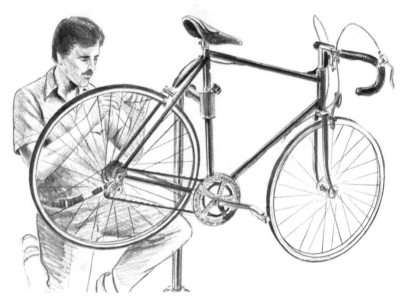

If all you ever hope to do is ride around the block on level terrain, you probably don't need ten gears. But I assume that since you are reading this chapter, you are interested in going appreciable distances over varying terrain in order to develop and maintain a good level of physical fitness. If this is the case, you should consider using a ten-speed to help you enjoy your training bouts.

I am not suggesting that you throw out your single-speed or three-speed bicycle if it's in good working order and serves your needs. But, I am suggesting that you make sure it fits you properly before proceeding with the cycling workouts presented later in this chapter. If it's too small or too big for you, it will probably be uncomfortable to pedal. You should have your seat adjusted to fit your body so that there's a slight bend at the knee when one pedal is in the down position. This position allows you to take full advantage of the strength of the large muscles in your thighs. If you are uncertain about whether your bike is in good working condition and fits you properly, take it to a reputable repair shop and get it serviced before starting your cycling workouts.

Covering all the ins and outs of selecting and fitting a bicycle is a chapter in itself. We've given you just the basic information. So, we suggest you visit some of the reputable bike shops in your area and ask questions. You may wish to enroll in a bicycle class. The YM / YWCAs or other similar centers offer courses in cycling that provide not only good exercise but instruction in bicycle operation, repair, and maintenance. Learning how to tune, adjust, and repair your bike will lessen your dependence on a bike shop.

How To Bike and Where

Frankly, it takes plenty of skill and savvy to ride a bicycle effectively, especially a ten-speed. During your early training sessions, it is important that you realize the need to become skilled at operating your bicycle in an efficient and safe manner. As you become more experienced in riding, you will become aware of your increased ability to control your bike under all conditions. This means being able to brake properly, to turn corners, and to navigate in tight situations such as traffic and narrow pathways. It means developing an awareness of the actions of other users of the road, and a realization of your limitations and the limitations of your equipment. Until you are a practiced cyclist, it is neither wise nor safe to go into heavy traffic or onto steep or winding roads or to cycle for long distances. Eventually, a kind of symbiotic union between you and your bike will occur. This comes from practice and experience. In other words, you learn how to be a bike rider by riding your bike.

Bicycle accident statistics show conclusively that when there is a collision between a bicycle and a car, it's usually the cyclist who is at fault. Thus you must learn to anticipate trouble. For example, go slow where automobile traffic is heavy. Be alert for pot holes or litter on the roads. Hitting one of these could send you tumbling into the path of the car. Use common sense and good judgment and choose roads that are less traveled.

Regulating Your Cycling Intensity

To achieve a *training effect* with a bicycle you need to challenge your cardiorespiratory system properly. As a general rule, we have found that you must cycle almost twice as fast as you would run in order to produce the same exercise heart rate. Recently a local research project revealed an interesting comparison. Two young men jogging at a seven-minute-mile pace had heart rates measured at 150 to 160 beats per minute. When they later cycled over the same outdoor course, they had to ride at more than a 3½-minute-mile pace to record approximately the same heart rates. When a young woman jogged at a 12-minute-mile

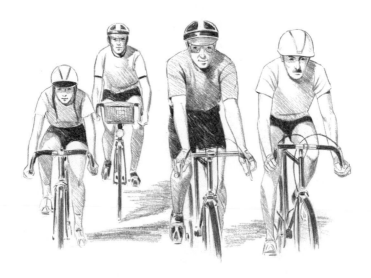

pace, her heart rate was 158. When she rode a bike, she had to ride at a five-minute-mile pace to reach a heart rate of 150, and a 4½-minute-mile pace to record a heart rate of 160. If you run or cycle at similar heart rates, you are, in theory, stressing your cardiorespiratory system to the same degree. Because of the smaller muscle mass used in cycling, the energy requirement (oxygen uptake) may be a little less than in running for the same heart rate. Nevertheless, when you can ride at a good pace long enough to stress the heart continuously and at a substantially elevated level (75% HR reserve), cycling can be an excellent form of exercise. The key is to develop the capability of pedaling vigorously to stress the heart and lungs adequately enough to achieve a training effect.

At this point, you may be wondering what pedaling gear you should use to attain a training effect. The mistake most people make is to pedal in too high a gear (heavy resistance). It is better to ride in a lower gear at a higher rpm (revolutions per minute) rather than in a higher gear at a lower rpm. At first you may want to count the number of complete turns you make with one pedal for one minute to better gauge your spinning rate. As a rule of thumb, spinning at 80 rpm in a gear that can be sustained reasonably well seems to work best.

If you have not been bicycling regularly, you should devote your early workouts to becoming familiar with riding a bike. The idea is to simply allow your body to break into the basics of riding a bike and to allow your body to adjust to the physical effort. Start out by riding for 10 to 20 minutes. In succeeding days, try to increase your total time, eventually working up to 30 minutes at a steady but comfortable pace. This is comparable to being able to walk two to three miles at a brisk pace. At first, don't be too concerned about how far you go or how fast you pedal. Concentrate on sustaining your riding effort and increasing your time or distance gradually. You may want to check your pulse at the end of your ride, but don't be too disturbed if it is not elevated to your target heart rate. Your main concern during the early stages of your cycling is to allow your muscles to become gradually accustomed to the pedaling and pumping motion. At first you may feel some soreness, but after a few days this should subside. Once you reach the point where you can ride non-stop at a comfortable pace for 30 minutes, you are ready to begin increasing your effort and attempting to ride at a more taxing and vigorous pace.

Avoiding Injuries

The most serious problem facing you when you cycle is the danger of falls or collisions and the injuries related to such accidents. Irvin Faria and Peter Cavanagh in their book the *Physiology and Biomechanics of Cycling* suggest serious skin abrasions can be best avoided by keeping your arms and legs covered. Of course in high, humid temperatures this suggestion may have to be somewhat modified in order to prevent heat problems. As mentioned earlier, a good precaution against head injuries from falls is to wear a helmet.

Pain commonly results from a bad riding position. Try to make some adjustments on the bike, such as adjusting the seat or handlebars. Changing handlebar height may help in your search for a pain-free riding position. Also, changing positions of your hands on the handlebars frequently during a long ride can help.

Saddle soreness can result from improper seat height. The material in your cycling pants can either cause or prevent minor irritations, boils, and blisters.

Pain in the joints, especially in the knee and ankle regions, can be caused by incorrect placement of the feet on the pedals and the distribution of force during the pedaling motion. Misalignment with the toe pointing in or out can lead to injury. Wearing proper footwear is crucial if you are to achieve pain-free cycling.

Muscular aches from cycling, as from any physical activity, will occur at times, but careful attention should be paid to joint pain. As we have stressed throughout this book, use good judgment and take things slowly at first. The charts that follow are geared to help you through the early stages and gradually progress to a higher level of physical fitness.

The Cycling Charts

If you have not been active in recent months, your first riding workouts should be at a relatively low or moderate speed. Start out by riding for 15 to 20 minutes. Repeat the next day, and then if you recover well within an hour after your riding bout, increase your ride the next day by five minutes. Gradually build up your riding time until you can ride for 30 minutes non-stop at a comfortable pace.

Now you are ready to get started. So refer to chart 1 and begin with step 1. This sequence of workouts is similar to the run-walk or swim-rest charts. They provide a simple approach for intensifying your cycling effort. Your own cycling tempo (pace) depends on your fitness and, of course, on your heart rate response to the cycling work. Step 1 calls for pedaling vigorously for three minutes. The key is to find the speed and gear at which you can maintain your training heart rate intensity and then use that pedaling speed. As you will note in chart 1, you repeat this segment (set) five more times for that day's workout. Repeat this workout the next session. If you are able to handle this amount of effort and recover favorably within an hour, add a set to the next workout (step 2, workout 3). Therefore, with every two workouts you add a set (three minutes vigorous cycling, one minute slow cycling) until you can do eight sets (step 3). Then you are ready to move to step 4, which calls for increasing your ride to four minutes, approximately ⅔ of a mile, before a recovery period of easy pedaling for one minute. Again, follow the pattern of increasing your number of sets with each step.

After you try out the suggested sets, you may need to adjust the cycling speed to provide a lesser or greater heart rate stimulus. Chart 2 provides steps for improving your fitness level. Eventually you will have achieved an endurance base and will be able to ride nine miles or more at your target heart rate (see step 10, chart 2). At this point, use your own judgment on the steps you take to reach continuous sessions of 30 minutes or more at your target heart rate. You can devise other workout variations that will be appropriate to your interests and needs. Long-distance touring trips (50 to 100 miles a day) are becoming popular pastimes during vacations or on weekends. Whether you tour on a bike or perform a series of timed repeats at 20-mph speeds, you will find the bicycle an excellent device for developing and maintaining physical fitness.

I think it's important to develop the habit of keeping a record of your cycling workouts. Such a record gives you a better idea of how you are doing, and it can assist you in learning about yourself and how you are responding to your workouts. A daily record can also be quite motivating. Become accustomed to making some general comments about your ride for that day. Note how far and how long you rode. Some days you may wish to include your weight, and in the early stages, recording your pulse rate will help you keep track of the intensity of your workouts and to make sound adjustments when needed. As your pulse levels off, it becomes less important to check it each day. Perhaps under unusual conditions, such as an extremely hot day or a very long ride, it would be worthwhile to note how hard your cardiorespiratory system was taxed. I enjoy keeping a weekly mileage chart. This provides systematic feed-back that helps me maintain my optimal fitness goals.

Many people like to make personal records. As one cyclist explains, "It's a chance to feel good and brag on paper instead of bending some-body's ear." Caution: Don't get carried away with trying to set a record each day. Many people use local races (running or biking) to strive for their personal records. Such a plan helps put more meaning into train-ing sessions. Let's face it, setting goals, whether they are improvements in your training bouts or racing events, can help to keep you motivated. The achievement of worthy goals can be satisfying.

Using the Cycling Charts

1. *Warm up with the stretching exercises* (Basic Twelve) to loosen and tone your main muscles groups. In like manner, cool down with some stretching exercises for about five to six minutes following your main cycling workout.

2. *For those who have been inactive* or who tested at a low-fitness level, your first two to three weeks of riding should be at moderate to low speeds with a gradual build-up of total distance each session. Start with bike rides of just 10 to 15 minutes. Gradually increase your time until you are capable of sustaining a comfortable and continuous ride of 30 minutes.

3. *When you can comfortably ride for 30 minutes* at a low speed, you are ready to begin with chart 1, which calls for a more vigorous intensity.

4. *The charts are arranged in steps.* A step represents two workouts, the second being a repeat of the first workout in that step. Providing you feel no adverse fatigue one hour after you have repeated the workout on the second day, you can move to the next step. If your cycling workout seems excessive, cut back to the previous step or continue repeating the workout you are on until you respond more favorably.

5. *The charts are designed so you will systematically* increase your number of cycling sets at your target heart rate. Start with three-minute rides with intermittent one-minute periods of easy cycling, with six repeats (step 1), and progress to four minutes and again strive to reach eight repeats. Remember not to fall into the trap of trying to increase your vigorous cycling workouts faster than the charts prescribe.

6. *As you progress through the charts,* you will reach the point where you can ride for ten minutes or more at your target heart rate intensity interspersed with short rest periods or easy pedaling.

7. *The charts are based on riding at a six-minute-mile pace (ten mph).* For some, this pace may not be adequate to elevate the heart rate to the target level. It is not uncommon to be able to work comfortably at your target heart rate at speeds closer to 3.5-to 5-minute-mile pace (12 to 17 mph). As you adapt to the cycling exercise you will most likely be able to ride faster and cover a greater total distance.

8. *You will note that the approximate workout time* ranges from 24 minutes to over 50 minutes of cycling. This amount of time is necessary if you are to achieve training changes comparable to running.

9. *Keep a record.* As you complete each workout session, check the appropriate box on the chart you are following. Also record your heart rate taken at the end of your last vigorous cycling set. Keeping an accurate record of your workouts helps you stay with it, and enables you to systematically follow your progress from day to day.

Chart #1 BICYCLE REPEATS

STEP	SESSION	MAXIMAL MET CAPACITY	THE WORKOUT VIGOROUS / SLOW CYCLING BOUTS	APPROXIMATE WORKOUT TIME (min.)	APPROXIMATE* DISTANCE OF VIGOROUS CYCLING (miles)	PEAK TRAINING HEART RATE	GENERAL COMMENTS
1	1☐ and 2☐	7	Cycle 3 min. at THR, then cycle easy or rest 1 min. (6X)	24	3.0		
2	3☐ and 4☐		Cycle 3 min. at THR, then cycle easy or rest 1 min. (7X)	28	3.5		
3	5☐ and 6☐	7.5	Cycle 3 min. at THR, then cycle easy or rest 1 min. (8X)	32	4.0		
4	7☐ and 8☐		Cycle 4 min. at THR, then cycle easy or rest 1 min. (6X)	30	2⅔		
5	9☐ and 10☐	8	Cycle 4 min. at THR, then cycle easy or rest 1 min. (7X)	35	3⅓		
6	11☐ and 12☐		Cycle 4 min. at THR, then cycle easy or rest 1 min. (8X)	40	4.0		
7	13☐ and 14☐	8.5	Cycle 5 min. at THR, then cycle easy or rest 1 min. (6X)	36	5.0		

Chart #1 BICYCLE REPEATS (cont'd)

THE WORKOUT

STEP	SESSION	MAXIMAL MET CAPACITY	VIGOROUS /SLOW CYCLING BOUTS	APPROXIMATE WORKOUT TIME (min.)	APPROXIMATE* DISTANCE OF VIGOROUS CYCLING (miles)	PEAK TRAINING HEART RATE	GENERAL COMMENTS
8	15 ☐ and 16 ☐		Cycle 5 min. at THR, then cycle easy or rest 1 min. (7X)	42	6.0		
9	17 ☐ and 18 ☐	9	Cycle 5 min. at THR, then cycle easy or rest 1 min. (8X)	48	6.5		
10	19 ☐ and 20 ☐		Cycle for 10 to 12 min. at THR, then cycle easy for 2 min. (3X)	36	6.0		

*Actual distance will depend on your cycling speed. The mileage estimated is based on a six-minute-mile (ten mph) pace. Some people may need to ride faster to achieve their target heart rate.

Chart #2 BICYCLING REPEATS

THE WORKOUT

STEP	SESSION	MAXIMAL MET CAPACITY	VIGOROUS-SLOW CYCLING BOUTS	APPROX. WORKOUT TIME (min.)	APPROXIMATE* DISTANCE OF VIGOROUS CYCLING (miles)	PEAK TRAINING HEART RATE	GENERAL COMMENTS
1	1 ☐ and 2 ☐	9.5	Cycle 8 min. at THR, cycle easy for 1 min. (3X) Cycle 10 min. at THR (1X)	37	5.5 to 6		
2	3 ☐ and 4 ☐		Cycle 8 min. at THR, cycle easy for 1 min. (2X) Cycle 10 min. at THR, cycle (2X)	40	6		
3	5 ☐ and 6 ☐	10.0	Cycle 8 min. at THR, cycle easy for 1 min. (1X) Cycle 10 min. at THR, cycle (3X)	42	6. 6.5		
4	7 ☐ and 8 ☐		Cycle 10 min. at THR, cycle easy for 1 min. (3X) Cycle 12 min. at THR, cycle easy for 1 min. (1X)	45	7		
5	9 ☐ and 10 ☐	10.5	Cycle 12 min. at THR, cycle easy for 1 min. (2X) Cycle 14 min. at THR, cycle (1X)	40	6 to 6.5		

THE WORKOUT

STEP	SESSION	MAXIMAL MET CAPACITY	VIGOROUS–SLOW CYCLING BOUTS	APPROX. WORKOUT TIME (min.)	APPROXIMATE* DISTANCE OF VIGOROUS CYCLING (miles)	PEAK TRAINING HEART RATE	GENERAL COMMENTS
6	11 □ and 12 □		Cycle 12 min. at THR, cycle easy for 1 min.(1X) Cycle 14 min. at THR, cycle easy for 1 min. (2X)	42	6 to 6.5		
7	13 □ and 14 □	11.0	Cycle 14 min. at THR, cycle easy for 1 min. (2X) Cycle 16 min. at THR (1X)	46	7 to 7.5		
8	15 □ and 16 □		Cycle 14 min.a t THR, cycle easy for 1 min. (1X) Cycle 16 min. at THR, cycle (2X)	48	7.5 to 8		
9	17 □ and 18 □	12.0	Cycle 16 min. at THR, cycle easy for 1 min. (2X) Cycle 18 min. at THR, cycle easy for 1 min. (1X)	52	8 to 8.5		
10	19 □ and 20 □		Cycle 18 min. at THR, cycle easy for 1 min. (3X)	56	9		

*Actual distance will depend on your cycling speed. The mileage estimated is based on a six-minute-mile (ten mph) pace. Some people may need to ride faster to achieve their target heart rate.

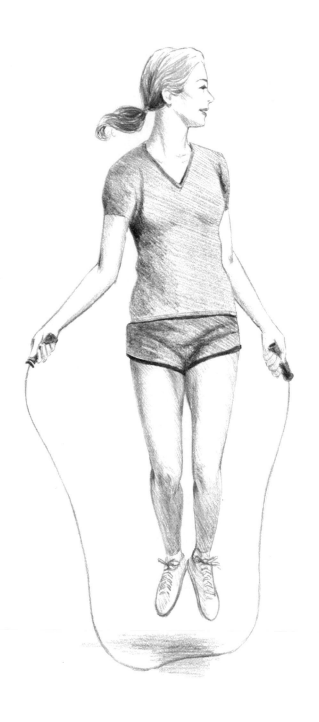

chapter twelve

Other Possibilities for Cardiorespiratory Fitness

Up to now we have dealt extensively with the four basic aerobic activities (walking, running, swimming, and cycling) for developing cardiorespiratory fitness. As long as you remember the principles for evaluating an activity must involve the large muscles of the body and be performed vigorously, continuously, and rhythmically — you shouldn't have problems evaluating other types of activities for your fitness training.

In this chapter we will first cover some specifics for using indoor equipment, followed by some insights on rope skipping and aerobic dance as fitness developers.

Indoor Fitness Equipment

During 1980, Americans spent almost $200 million on indoor fitness equipment ranging from $3 for a jump rope to $2,000 for a sleek stationary bicycle to as much as $8,000 for a motorized treadmill. Not only have these exercise tools become more common in the home, but many corporations are now developing exercise rooms with a variety of exercise devices for their employees. Exercise centers equipped with exercise bikes, rowing machines, treadmills, and massive fitness machines are opening in almost every city and town.

There are dozens of exercise devices on the market today, but many are useless for developing and maintaining physical fitness. Dr. William Haskell, an exercise physiologist in preventive medicine at Stanford University Medical School, observed candidly, "Many people buy a home exercise device hoping that it will make exercising easy.

217

When it doesn't happen that way, the item ends up in the basement or a closet."

If you decide you wish to use a home exercise device, make sure it will help you attain and maintain optimal fitness. You should select equipment that allows you to exercise most of the large muscles of your body continuously and rhythmically. Such exercise, if rigorous enough, expends calories, helps increase endurance and muscle tone, and aids cardiorespiratory fitness development.

Of course, if you are to get the most out of these added approaches to exercise, each activity must follow the basic guidelines of intensity, frequency, and duration as previously discussed in this book. In order to improve in cardiorespiratory and muscular fitness, a vigorous over-load is necessary in all conditioning programs.

Exercise equipment that provides a vigorous challenge to the body might be just what is needed for some people to get started. And many of these devices provide a reasonable alternative or diversion for the walker, runner, swimmer, or cyclist.

In the following section we discuss some of the better home devices and provide suggestions on how to use such equipment effectively. By applying the basic principles described in the previous chapters, you will see how easy it is to adapt your workouts to using indoor equip-ment.

The Stationary Bicycle

For many people the stationary exercise bike with adjustable pedal resistance is a convenient means for daily exercise. For those who are unable to run because of orthopedic problems, the exercise bike is an excellent alternative for providing an adequate stimulus for the heart and circulation. We use the bike in our fitness program at Ball State as a back-up to our walking and running workouts. When an injury begins to hinder a participant's workout, we substitute bike exercises for a few days to help them keep up with their program. For those who do not wish to run or walk in public and prefer the privacy of exercising in their home, riding a stationary bike is the best alternative. Some peo-ple listen to the stereo, watch television, or even read a book to help pass the time as they pedal toward fitness.

It is quite easy to develop a program using a stationary bike if you understand the principles behind the run-walk-run method of train-ing. (See Chapter 9). The same standards apply to training on a stationary bike. Basically you ride repeated segments of resistance pedaling with short rest periods of no-resistance pedaling or walking around the room. Each workout can be gradually intensified by increasing the length and number of the riding sets as you begin to get in shape.

A good stationary exercise bicycle (often referred to as a bicycle ergometer) should measure the amount of work being performed as you pedal against a known amount of resistance. However, many stationary bicycles on the market do not accurately measure the amount of work being performed. Although much cheaper to purchase than a calibrated bicycle ergometer, they leave much to be desired for the serious exerciser.

Before getting into the specifics of using the bicycle ergometer, let's explain how it works. A bicycle ergometer is constructed so that a braking mechanism on a large flywheel can be regulated to provide friction. This friction is measured in specific amounts. The gearing mechanism and the wheel diameter are constructed so that one full rotation of the pedals moves a point on the wheel an exact distance. On a Monark bicycle the distance is six meters and on a Tunturi bike the distance is three meters. Therefore, if you know the pedal revolutions per minute, the distance traveled can be determined and, if you know the amount of friction being applied, you can determine the workload.

Generally, pedal speeds in the range of 50 to 60 rpm provide a good pedaling tempo. The workload settings are expressed in terms of force times distance, such as kilopond meters or kilogram meters, depending on the manufacturer. Instructions that come with the bike will help you determine workloads and show you how to set the workload at a level

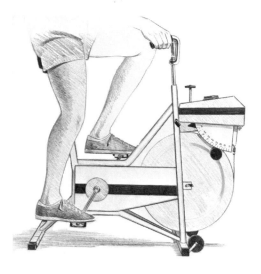

that will stress your heart and lungs enough to reach your target heart rate. Knowing how to set the numbers is all you need to know to regulate the resistance on the bike.

The importance of being able to regulate the workload accurately becomes quite evident as you exercise from day to day. When you follow a systematic pattern of exercise workouts, you want to be able to come back the next session to a device that can reproduce workloads similar or slightly heavier than the previous day. The better the bike, the easier it is to regulate your workouts and follow a systematic program of exercise.

If your bike is not calibrated, you can still use it by measuring your heart rate either during your pedaling or immediately after. This helps you regulate the intensity of your effort. The key is to work at your target heart rate whether your bike is calibrated or non-calibrated.

Selecting a bike. As the saying goes, "You get what you pay for." This is especially true in purchasing a bicycle ergometer. You don't necessarily need the top of the line, but you do need a bike with quality construction. Look for a sturdy bike weighing around 45 to 55 pounds. The flywheel on these models should be weighted, balanced, and calibrated. The seat should be sturdy and adjustable. You can definitely notice a smoother ride as you pedal the better-quality bikes. They will hold up well under heavy usage and provide accurately measured and reproducible workloads. With a quality instrument, you will have greater control over the progression of your workouts and will be able to advance properly.

Some considerations before starting. The principles of warming up (Chapter 7) and the guidelines for regulating intensity (Chapter 4) should be applied when using the stationary bike. Remember, your goal is to increase gradually the amount of exercise you can do over a period of weeks, keeping well within your physical capabilities. The idea is to stimulate your heart, enabling it to beat near your target heart rate.

In the privacy of your home, what you wear when you work out on a stationary bike is simply up to you. You need shoes; running shoes will do. Shorts with some thickness in the seat to prevent saddle sores are recommended, or perhaps a fluffy towel across the seat will suffice.

As mentioned earlier, you may want to watch TV or listen to the stereo while cycling. However, you are going to perspire (most likely profusely), so plan accordingly if you want to prevent your carpet or flooring from becoming soaked with sweat. Your basement, utility room, or garage may be the best place for your regular exercise work-outs on the bike.

To become accustomed to your bike, we suggest you pedal for a few days without setting the resistance. Try to pedal at a cadence of one pedal revolution per second, or 60 rpm. If you respond will to this brief introduction, set the resistance up a little and check to see if your exercise effort is challenging enough to elevate your heart rate to a reasonable target for your level of fitness. The following charts (1 through 4) are similar to the run-walk charts in Chapter 9. Instead of running, you pedal at a workload heavy enough to elevate to your target heart rate. You adjust the workload by tightening the mechanical friction to increase the resistance.

If you find it extremely taxing to pedal an ergometer set with some resistance, turn to Chapter 8 and adapt the walking charts to your needs. For example, chart 1, step 1 (page 222) calls for 15 to 20 minutes minutes of steady walking. Instead, cycle with no resistance for 15 to 20 minutes. Increase this effort by four minutes every two workouts. Once you can sustain 44 minutes of cycling without resistance, then return to this chapter and try the stationary cycling ride-rest charts. Begin at chart 1, step 1.

If you're using the bike as an alternative to running, try to duplicate the time and intensity of your run-walk or running program. Even if you have been running continuously for 20 to 30 minutes, you may have to allow yourself some brief rest intervals until you become accustomed to the leg-muscle fatigue that accompanies the early training period with a bike.

Before you start your workout, make sure the seat is properly adjusted. There should be a slight bend at the knee when your toes are on the pedal in the fully down position

Keep a record of your progress and monitor your heart rate to be sure you are putting out enough effort. Your goal is to eventually be able to pedal for 30 minutes or more at your target heart rate at least four times a week. As you strive for this goal you will begin to realize the good feeling that is part of being physically fit.

The Rowing Machine

A rowing machine allows you to stimulate the actual work of rowing a boat. It consists of a seat that moves forward and back on a metal frame as you provide the rowing movements with two short oars. You can ad-

Chart #1 STATIONARY CYCLING STARTER PROGRAM

THE WORKOUT

STEP	SESSION	MAXIMAL MET CAPACITY	NO RESISTANCE PEDALING (min.)	RIDE-RESTS	NO RESISTANCE PEDALING (min.)	TOTAL WORKOUT TIME (min.)	PEAK TRAINING HEART RATE	GENERAL COMMENTS
1	1☐ and 2☐	7	20	ride 30 sec. and rest 30 sec. (4X)	10	33.5		
2	3☐ and 4☐		17.5	ride 30 sec. and rest 30 sec. (6X)	10	33.0		
3	5☐ and 6☐		15	ride 30 sec. and rest 30 sec. (6X) ride 45 sec. and rest 40 sec. (2X)	8	31.0		
4	7☐ and 8☐		15	ride 45 sec. and rest 30 sec. (4X) ride 1 min. and rest 30 sec. (2X)	8	30.5		
5	9☐ and 10☐		12	ride 45 sec. and rest 30 sec. (4X) ride 1 min. and rest 30 sec. (3X)	8	29.0		
6	11☐ and 12☐	7.5	12	ride 45 sec. and rest 30 sec. (4X) ride 1 min. and rest 30 sec. (4X)	8	30.5		
7	13☐ and 14☐		10	ride 45 sec. and rest 30 sec. (2X) ride 1 min. and rest 30 sec. (5X)	6	27.0		

Chart #1 STATIONARY CYCLING
STARTER PROGRAM (cont'd)

STEP	SESSION	MAXI-MAL MET CAPA-CITY	NO RESISTANCE PEDALING (min.)	THE WORKOUT RIDE-RESTS	NO RESISTANCE PEDALING (min.)	TOTAL WORKOUT TIME (min.)	PEAK TRAIN-ING HEART RATE	GENERAL COMMENTS
8	15 ☐ and 16 ☐	7.5	10	ride 45 sec. and rest 30 sec. (2X) ride 1 min. and rest 30 sec. (6X)	6	29.5		
9	17 ☐ and 18 ☐		10	ride 45 sec. and rest 30 sec. (2X) ride 1 min. and rest 30 sec. (7X)	6	30.0		
10	19 ☐ and 20 ☐		10	ride 45 sec. and rest 30 sec. (2X) ride 1 min. and rest 30 sec. (8X)	6	31.5		

Chart #2 STATIONARY CYCLING INTERMEDIATE PROGRAM

STEP	SESSION	MAXIMAL MET CAPACITY	NO RESISTANCE PEDALING (min.)	THE WORKOUT RIDE-RESTS	NO RESISTANCE PEDALING (min.)	TOTAL WORKOUT TIME (min.)	PEAK TRAINING HEART RATE	GENERAL COMMENTS
1	1 ☐ and 2 ☐	8	10	ride 1 min. and rest 30 sec. (8X) / ride 1.5 min. and rest 45 sec. (2X)	4	28		
2	3 ☐ and 4 ☐		10	ride 1 min. and rest 30 sec. (6X) / ride 1.5 min. and rest 45 sec. (4X)	4	28		
3	5 ☐ and 6 ☐		8	ride 1 min. and rest 30 sec. (5X) / ride 1.5 min. and rest 45 sec. (4X) / ride 2 min. (1X)	4	30		
4	7 ☐ and 8 ☐		8	ride 1 min. and rest 30 sec. (2X) / ride 1.5 min. and rest 45 sec. (6X) / ride 2 min. and rest 1 min. (2X)	4	32		
5	9 ☐ and 10 ☐		6	ride 1 min. and rest 30 sec. (2X) / ride 1.5 min. and rest 45 sec. (4X) / ride 2 min. and rest 1 min. (4X)	4	33		

Chart # 2 STATIONARY CYCLING
INTERMEDIATE PROGRAM (cont'd)

STEP	SESSION	MAXI-MAL MET CAPA-CITY	NO RESISTANCE PEDALING (min.)	THE WORKOUT RIDE-RESTS	NO RESISTANCE PEDALING (min.)	TOTAL WORKOUT TIME (min.)	PEAK TRAIN-ING HEART RATE	GENERAL COMMENTS
6	11 ☐ and 12 ☐	8.5	6	ride 1 min. and rest 30 sec. (2X) ride 1.5 min. and rest 45 sec. (2X) ride 2 min. and rest 1 min. (6X)	4	33		
7	13 ☐ and 14 ☐		4	ride 1.5 min. and rest 30 sec. (2X) ride 2 min. and rest 45 sec. (7X)	4	32		
8	15 ☐ and 16 ☐		4	ride 1.5 min. and rest 30 sec. (8X) ride 2 min. and rest 45 sec. (8X)	2	32		
9	17 ☐ and 18 ☐		2	ride 2 min. and rest 30 sec. (8X) ride 3 min. and rest 1 min. (2X)	2	30		
10	19 ☐ and 20 ☐		2	ride 2 min. and rest 30 sec. (6X) ride 3 min. and rest 1 min. (4X)	2	34		

Chart #3 STATIONARY CYCLING
ADVANCED PROGRAM

STEP	SESSION	MAXMIMAL MET CAPACITY	THE WORKOUT			
			RIDE-RESTS	TOTAL RIDING TIME (min.)	PEAK TRAINING HEART RATE	GENERAL COMMENTS
1	1☐ and 2☐	9	ride 2 min. rest 30 sec. (5X) ride 3 min. rest 1 min. (5X)	25		
2	3☐ and 4☐		ride 2 min. rest 30 sec. (3X) ride 3 min. rest 1 min. (4X) ride 4 min. rest 2 min. (2X)	26		
3	5☐ and 6☐		ride 3 min. rest 1 min. (4X) ride 4 min. rest 2 min. (3X)	24		
4	7☐ and 8☐		ride 3 min. rest 1 min. (3X) ride 4 min. rest 2 min. (4X)	25		
5	9☐ and 10☐		ride 3 min. rest 1 min. (2X) ride 4 min. rest 1.5 min. (2X) ride 5 min. rest 2 min. (2X)	24		
6	11☐ and 12☐	10	ride 4 min. rest 1.5 min. (2X) ride 5 min. rest 2 min. (2X) ride 6 min. (1X)	24		

Chart #3 STATIONARY CYCLING
ADVANCED PROGRAM (cont'd)

THE WORKOUT

STEP	SESSION	MAXMIMAL MET CAPACITY	RIDE-RESTS	TOTAL RIDING TIME (min.)	PEAK TRAINING HEART RATE	GENERAL COMMENTS
7	13 ☐ and 14 ☐	10	ride 4 min. rest 1 min. (2X) ride 8 min. rest 2.5 min. (2X)	24		
8	15 ☐ and 16 ☐		ride 4 min. rest 1 min. (2X) ride 10 min. rest 2.5 min. (1X) ride 6 min. (1X)	24		
9	17 ☐ and 18 ☐		ride 4 min. rest 1 min. (1X) ride 10 min. rest 2 min. (2X)	24		
10	19 ☐ and 20 ☐		ride 20 min.	20		

Chart #4 STATIONARY CYCLING
ADVANCED TO MAINTENANCE

THE WORKOUT

STEP	SESSION	RIDE-RESTS	TOTAL TIME (min.)	PEAK TRAINING HEART RATE	GENERAL COMMENTS
1	Mon. ☐	ride for 20 to 24 min. rest 2-min. ride for 5 to 6 min.	25–30		
2	Tue. ☐	ride for 15 to 18 min. rest 2 min. ride for 10 to 12 min.	25–30		
3	Thur. ☐	ride for 25 to 30 min.	25–30		
	Fri. ☐	ride for 15 to 18 min.	15–18		
5	Mon. ☐	ride for 20 to 24 min. rest 2-4 min. ride for 5 to 6 min. rest 1 min. ride for 5 to 6 min.	30–36		
6	Tue. ☐	ride for 15 to 18 min. rest 2-3 min. ride for 15 to 18 min	30–36		
7	Thur. ☐	ride for 30 to 36 min.	30–36		
8	Fri. ☐	ride for 25 to 30 min.	25–30		

Chart #4 STATIONARY CYCLING
ADVANCED TO MAINTENANCE (cont'd)

THE WORKOUT

STEP	SESSION	RIDE-RESTS	TOTAL TIME (min.)	PEAK TRAINING HEART RATE	GENERAL COMMENTS
9	Mon. ☐	ride for 25 to 30 min. rest 2–4 min. ride for 10 to 12 min.	35–42		
10	Tue. ☐	ride for 20 to 24 min. rest 2–3 min. ride for 15 to 18 min.	35–42		
11	Thur. ☐	ride for 35 to 42 min.	35–42		
12	Fri. ☐	ride for 30 to 36 min.	30–36		

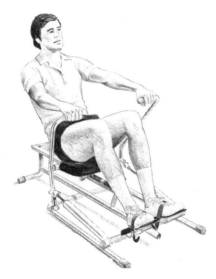

just the resistance to suit your strength and endurance capabilities. The Tunturi rowing machine has a continuous braking resistance for each of the two oars. A rowing machine can do much for strengthening your arms and back muscles. It is also good for the abdominal muscles. Because this versatile machine allows you to exercise most of the large muscles of the body continuously and rhythmically, it can provide a good stimulus to the cardiorespiratory system. Using a rowing machine at the proper intensity can help burn calories, increase your endurance, and improve your muscle tone.

If you wish to follow a systematic chart while using a rowing machine, refer to the bicycle charts in Chapter 11 and follow that sequential pattern. It's important to start out at the proper point. Chapter 5 will assist you in determining your maximal MET capacity and your present physical status. Then, refer to the charts in Chapter 11 and set the workload so you can work at your target heart rate.

The Treadmill

We have previously discussed the treadmill (Chapter 5) as a means of testing your fitness, but these devices can also be useful for exercise training. There are two types; non-motorized and motorized. If you have access to a motorized treadmill, you have an excellent device for

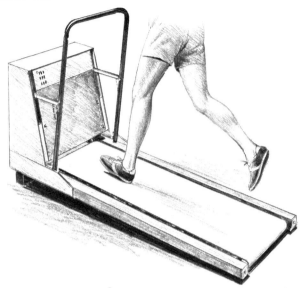

walking and running. The charts in Chapter 8 and 9 adapt easily to treadmill training. The big disadvantage of a motorized treadmill is the initial cost and operating expense. The one we use in our laboratory cost over $9,000. However, some inexpensive motorized treadmills cost as little as $2,000. The less expensive models cannot be inclined to increase the workload, a necessity when testing for maximal METS, but this is not needed when you are training. The non-motorized and even less costly treadmill operates with rollers under the belt that moves as you walk. You actually become the motor. If walking and running at home is your desire, a treadmill can be a worthwhile device for you. Refer to the Run-Walk charts in Chapter 9 if you wish to follow a systematic plan of training using the treadmill.

The Indoor Jogger

"Indoor jogging" is being promoted as "trauma-reduced aerobic exercise." The early reports on the effectiveness of this small trampoline-type apparatus for getting and keeping in shape is not too encouraging.

I recently had a chance to work out on the indoor jogger as part of a research study. With this apparatus, you run in place on a rubberized trampoline surface. The surface provides a consistent and resilient running platform. The claims are that it reduces the stress on the ankles, knees, and legs that often comes from running on a hard surface. Again you need to elevate your heart rate to the proper target level by the

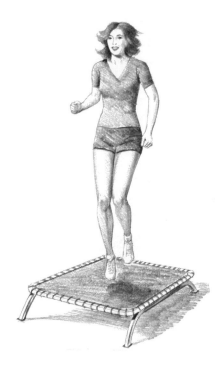

speed of your running movements. For some of us in the study this was difficult, even when we lifted our knees high and increased our running tempo. It appears this device may be effective for some people starting out, but the problem of being able to elevate your heart rate to a good stimulus level could be a problem.

Dr. Victor Katch and his associates at the University of Michigan tend to agree with our observation. Recently they published a research study that examined the energy cost and heart rate response of "rebound-running" on the indoor jogger. Their findings indicated an average intensity of five METs and heart rates averaging 116 beats a minute. This placed the activity in the low- to moderate-exercise category for the subjects tested. Although the subjects enjoyed the rebound-running, they stated that they were not able to feel the same training stimulus as when they jog. Doctor Katch infers that some of the previous claims made by the manufacturers of the indoor joggers as to the beneficial changes in maximal oxygen uptake should be viewed with suspicion. Keep in mind, for rebound-running to be effective as a cardiorespiratory conditioner, the intensity must be near your target heart rate.

Rope Skipping

Despite recent claims by jump-rope enthusiasts, rope skipping is no more magical than any other fitness program. When you consider the claims made about rope skipping, no wonder sales of jump ropes have skyrocketed. "It doesn't cost much," "Anyone can do it," "You can do it anywhere," "It can produce the greatest amount of conditioning in the shortest amount of time": such statements certainly appeal to the person seeking a way to become physically fit. However, our own research conducted in the Human Performance Laboratory at Ball State University and other recent studies question some of these claims. For sure, skipping rope is an excellent activity for agility and coordination. Besides, it's fun! Nevertheless, rope skipping for fitness has to be vigorous. In addition, it takes time to achieve optimal benefits, and as with other fitness activities, if you do too much, too soon, you can easily injure yourself. For rope skipping to be an effective mode of fitness training, you must work at a substantial intensity, sustain this intensity long enough, and do it regularly. Just as in walking, running, swimming, or cycling, the effectiveness of your exercise workouts for increasing your fitness depends on your capability to work at your target heart rate and sustain it.

When starting out on a fitness program, whether it's rope skipping or running, the same precautions hold true. Start slowly and at a level of exertion well within your abilities. Our intention is to show you how to set up a program of rope skipping that is reasonable and safe. But first let's consider how the body responds to rope skipping and how skipping rope compares to other fitness modes.

An often-quoted study makes the claim that ten minutes of rope skipping is equivalent to 30 minutes of running. To the individual searching for a convenient and inexpensive form of exercise, this seems like good news. Unfortunately, it is nonsense! Some basic physiological facts contradict such a claim. For example, most runners can burn at least ten calories per minute while running (some even go as high as 15 calories). For a 30-minute period, that's 300 calories. Now, to jump rope for ten minutes and burn 300 calories means that you must burn 30 calories per minute. Such a value is unrealizable. Most highly trained endurance runners cannot sustain 30 calories of energy for even a few minutes. When the marathoner Bill Rodgers was tested at our Human Performance Laboratory, his energy cost for running at a

5:37-mile pace was approximately 15 calories/minute. His maximal energy expenditure at exhaustion was only 22.7 calories/minute.

Skipping rope does raise the heart rate substantially. However, the energy expenditure (calories/minute), when comparisons are made at the same heart rate, are not as high as the requirements for running. When performed at the same heart rate intensity, running requires more energy (calories) than skipping rope. The reason for this appears to be that more of the total body is involved in running than in skipping rope. Therefore, the runner burns more calories at the same heart rate. If a person wants to get physiological training benefits from rope skipping, it appears that heart rate intensity and the time spent skipping have to be at least as great as running.

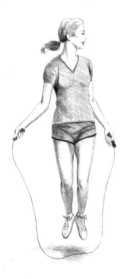

More research is needed to assess the long-term training benefits of regular workouts of rope skipping. Furthermore, the energy requirement imposed by skipping rope (even at a low 80 turns per minute) is not reasonable for the adult who has been inactive. For example, our observations and the findings of others suggest that the metabolic rate (energy cost) for skipping rope is about eight to ten times the resting rate (eight to ten METS). This represents a rather strenuous activity and a level of exertion that is near maximal or maximal for the majority of adults beginning a fitness program. We have observed that the heart rate for out-of-shape people reaches close to maximal with only 30 to 60 seconds of continuous jumping. A go-slow approach is reasonable for rope skipping.

Some Considerations Before Starting

If you want to try skipping as a means of training, you need a good rope. It should be long enough to reach from armpit to armpit while passing under both feet. The models with plastic disks that slide around the rope provide a good balance and weight to the rope. Handles that are reasonably weighted will keep the rope from getting tangled.

If you haven't skipped before, you need to learn how to turn the rope, to jump rhythmically, and put the two together. To get accustomed to turning the rope, place both handles (ends of the rope) in the same hand. Twirl the rope from back to front parallel to your side. As it circles let the loop hit the floor lightly. Your hand should make a circle of four to eight inches in diameter. Do about 50 to 60 turns then change hands and do it again.

To understand skipping styles, four basic terms need to be defined: (1) A *jump* refers to taking off on both feet and landing on both feet; (2) a *hop* refers to taking off on one foot and landing on the same foot; (3) a *leap* refers to taking off on one foot and landing on the other; and (4) a *rebound* refers to the smaller jump that follows a two-footed jump.

Now we suggest you learn the two-foot jump with rebound. Without the rope, jump into the air high enough for an imaginary rope to slide under your feet. Land on the balls of your feet. This is followed by a second jump (rebound), but of minimal height. During the rebound your knees bend more. You can count—jump on *one* and rebound on *two*. (The two-foot jump without a rebound or the single-foot hop or a leaping style are other variations you can try after you have mastered the two-foot jump with rebound.)

Now combine the one-hand turn and the two-foot jump with rebound. Listen to the rhythm of the rope striking the floor as you twirl it. Then begin to jump in time with the rhythm of the rope allowing a rebound in between each jump and strike. After 15 to 20 twirls, change hands and try the other side.

When you are comfortable with the one-hand turn with jump and rebound you are ready to try the two-hand jump. Start with the rope's loop lying behind your heels on the floor. Each hand holds a handle lightly. Your arms are extended forward. To get the rope turning, swing the extended arms down and back and as you feel the rope rise bring your hands toward your hips in a circular manner.

Don't be upset if you don't succeed at first. Turning the rope effectively is a skill that must be acquired. After you make the first turn keep your elbows closer to your sides. The hands are in front of your hips and your forearms relaxed. Your body should be erect but relaxed. Look straight ahead, not down at your feet. Learn to make small circles with the hands as you turn the rope. Eventually you will get the feel of the rope. Then begin thinking about making a soft landing after each jump.

If you are out of shape, start slowly and do not do too much, too soon. In fact, we recommend that you first be capable of walking a brisk three miles before you begin a rope skipping program. Be sure to warm up with the stretching exercises in Chapter 7. During your warm-up, include some running and jumping in place. This will help your body get loose and warm.

Jumping rope places a sudden and rigorous demand on the ankle, knee, and hip joints. Even people who can run for 30 minutes have difficulty jumping for ten minutes because of the constant force on the legs. However, it isn't the aerobic requirement (calories used) that tires them, rather it is the acute stress on the leg muscles that limits their effectiveness.

A rope-skipping routine is presented in chart 5.(p. 238) It is based on the same principles of all the suggested exercise charts in this book. During the early steps we suggest brief segments of skipping separated by short rest intervals. At first the workout sets may seem too easy. But beware! Gradually, the length and number of sets will increase, and you will begin to experience the vigorous exertion of rope skipping.

The routines are designed to help you progress to sustaining three ten-minute sets of skipping. We recommend a rate of 80 turns (one turn equals a jump and rebound while the rope revolves once) per minute. This rate of skipping will tend to provide a heart rate elevation close to the recommended training heart rate (75% HR reserve). For some of you, a lessening of the rate of rope turns may be necessary. As you acquire skill, you may need to increase the rate of rope turns or your style (hops, leaps, or combinations) to maintain your training heart rate. For those who are in reasonably good physical condition, starting out on step 3 or 4 shown in chart 5 may be preferred. For those who have been inactive, repeating the previous day's workout may be necessary. The key is to progress slowly and avoid unnecessary soreness and injuries. You should feel fully recovered an hour after your jumping session.

Aerobic Dance

The popularity of aerobic dance has swept the country due, in part, to Jacki Sorensen, who is credited as the innovator of aerobic dance. It involves total body movement to peppy music. Some describe it as looking like an amateur musical performance. Jacki Sorensen and others have choreographed many routines that involve walking, running, hopping, skipping, and various arm swings and kicking movements. The key to this popular activity is that it is fun. Many people (mostly women) wouldn't exercise if they didn't dance. The only attire needed is running apparel — good shoes, shorts, and T-shirt. Another important aspect is that the routines can be adapted to your fitness capabilities. Dancers can work at low, moderate, or high intensity levels to the same music. One thing stressed by Jacki Sorensen is that you must keep moving continuously for 35 to 45 minutes. Thus one can walk through the routines of dance vigorously. Participants are taught to monitor their own heart rates in order to assure they are near their target heart beat. A properly choreographed routine can require a complete use of every muscle of the body. Good muscle flexibility is involved and cardiorespiratory benefits are possible. As usual, the intensity, duration and frequency of your dance periods determine the benefits. Regular and vigorous dancing can be a good fitness activity. In addition, the release of emotional and mental tension through self-expression to music is a bonus.

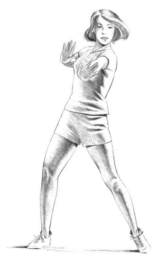

Chart #5 ROPE SKIPPING
(AT 80 ROPE TURNS PER MINUTE)

STEP	SESSION	THE WORKOUT SKIPS–RESTS	TOTAL JUMPING TIME (Approximate min.)
1	1 ☐ 2 ☐ 3 ☐ 4 ☐	Start with six 20-second bouts with a ten second rest interval between each. On each succeeding workout add two sets until you can do twelve sets; then go to the next step.	2–4
2	5 ☐ 6 ☐ 7 ☐ 8 ☐	Start with six 30-second bouts with a ten second rest interval between each. On each succeeding workout add two sets until you can do twelve; then go to the next step.	3–6
3	9 ☐ 10 ☐ 11 ☐ 12 ☐ 13 ☐	Start with six 45-second bouts with a 15-second rest interval between each. On each succeeding workout add one set until you can do ten sets; then go to the next step.	4.5–7.5
4	14 ☐ 15 ☐ 16 ☐ 17 ☐ 18 ☐	Start with six one-minute bouts with a 30-second rest interval between each. On each succeeding workout add one set until you can do ten sets; then go on to the next step.	6–10

Chart #5 ROPE SKIPPING
(AT 80 ROPE TURNS PER MINUTE) (cont'd)

STEP	SESSION	SKIPS–RESTS	TOTAL JUMPING TIME (Approximate min.)
5	19 20 21 22 23 ☐ ☐ ☐ ☐ ☐	Start with four two-minute bouts with a 30-second rest interval between each. On each succeeding workout add one set until you can do eight sets; then go to the next step.	8–16
6	24 25 26 27 28 ☐ ☐ ☐ ☐ ☐	Start with four three-minute bouts with a 30-second rest interval between each. On each succeeding workout add one set until you can do eight sets; then go on to the next step.	12–24
7	29 30 31 32 33 ☐ ☐ ☐ ☐ ☐	Start with four four-minute bouts with a 30-second rest interval between each. On each succeeding workout add one set until you can do eight sets; then go on to the next step.	16–32
8	34 35 36 37 38 39 40 ☐ ☐ ☐ ☐ ☐ ☐ ☐	Try to sustain skipping for ten minutes, then rest for two or three minutes. Repeat. On each succeeding workout try to skip comfortably for as long as you can, up to 10 minutes. Eventually your goal is to complete three ten-minute bouts of skipping.	10–30

Studies have shown that routines can stimulate the body's energy systems adequately. For example, moderate-intensity sessions compare to walking at 3.5 mph (about a 17-minute-mile pace), whereas a high intensity routine that involves some running is comparable to running at 5.5 mph (about 11-minute-mile pace). To put it another way, the energy requirements can range upward from four to five calories to around nine to ten calories a minute. The big advantage to aerobic dancing is that it is gradable at three intensity levels — low, moderate, or high. Also there is no embarrassment if you happen to get out of step with the others as long as you keep moving. The emphasis is on continuous rhythmical movement to stimulate your cardiorespiratory system.

Most YM / YWCAs and many private exercise facilities offer classes in aerobic dance. It is not difficult in most communities to enroll in such classes. Although most dancing is done in groups in public places with a leader, it seems reasonable that once a few routines are learned, you could dance in your own home. In fact, there are programs on television that allow you to dance with a leader and accompanying music.

I met Jacki Sorensen years ago when she was just beginning her aerobic dance classes. We were on the same program for the President's Council for Physical Fitness. She openly admitted to me that running was the best exercise and she averaged around 40 miles a week running. However, she realized then as many of us do now that running is not appealing for many people. Thus aerobic dancing may fill the exercise need for many. If they didn't dance, they wouldn't do anything!

Summary

Unfortunately, there are many self-proclaimed authorities feeding our lazy, automated society erroneous facts about home exercising. According to Dr. William Haskell, there seems to be an inverse relationship between the actual effectiveness of a particular device and the claims made about it. Distinguishing the good advice from the bad is one of the more difficult tasks for beginning exercisers. If you have read the previous chapters of this book and have been following one or more of the exercise charts, you now have the rudiments for understanding what it takes to get physically fit. As I've said all along, it takes effort to be physically fit. No machine can rub, vibrate, or whirlpool off your excess fat and get you in shape.

Your primary concern, regardless of what equipment or exercise mode you use, is to adhere to the guidelines of intensity, duration, and frequency as presented in this book. Be sure your workout is rhythmic and sustaining so you can realize a training effect. When you have found a program of exercise that suits you, keep at it. Starting out on an indoor fitness device, a jump rope, or with aerobic dance can serve as the catalyst to other fitness activities. As you gain confidence in your abilities and improve your fitness, you may wish to try other fitness ventures.

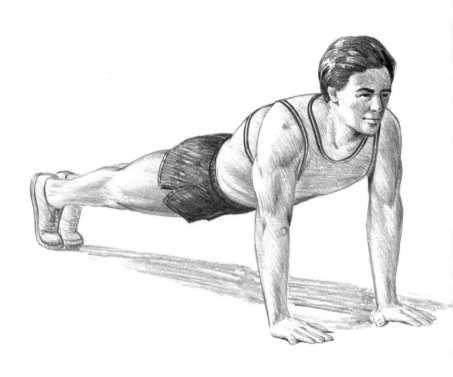

chapter thirteen

Developing Strength and Muscular Endurance

Why do you need strength and muscular endurance? First, strength and muscular endurance are valuable assets in many everyday activities. Having muscles that are reasonably toned, strong, and capable of easily enduring the strains of everyday tasks will undoubtedly make you more effective in your endeavors.

Second, low back pain, a common complaint of many men and women, can be helped with appropriate exercises that strengthen the muscles of the abdomen and trunk region. It is well documented that backaches generally result from muscles in the spinal region that are too weak to support the weight of the body. Common remedies for back pain, such as heat application, diathermy, or even medication, don't get at the primary cause — muscle weakness.

Third, whether you walk, run, swim, cycle, or play sports regularly, the chance for injury is always there. Many muscle pulls occur partly because of weakness in either the pulled muscle or its opposing muscle. You need proportional strength. For instance, runners tend to over-develop the back leg muscles, and the front muscles of the leg do not get adequate development. This can cause a muscular imbalance that may lead to injury. Therefore, these muscles need some strengthening to assure a better balance among the leg and thigh muscles. In addition, since walkers, runners, and even cyclists do not get enough arm and shoulder exercise, these body segments need specific strength and endurance exercises.

This chapter provides some basic exercises for strength and endurance development. Keep in mind, the idea is not to build large bulky muscles but to build muscles that can help you be effective in your everyday tasks or in your chosen recreation, whether it is gardening, rock hunting, backpacking, road racing, or golf. Therefore, you need

243

exercises that strengthen the major muscle groups as well as counteract muscle imbalances. Integration of such exercises into your chosen cardiorespiratory fitness program will prepare you more completely for optimal living.

Improving Strength and Endurance

Strength is the capacity of a muscle to exert force against a resistance. Endurance is the capacity of a muscle to exert force repeatedly over a period of time, or to apply strength and sustain it. It is beneficial not only to be able to apply force (strength), or to apply force with speed (power), but also to be able to sustain this force over a period of time (endurance).

There are two basic types of muscular contractions. *Isotonic* (dynamic) contractions shorten the muscles with a resulting motion, such as bending the arms as you lift a bag of groceries. *Isometric* (static) contractions are those in which the muscles apply force but their overall length does not change and movement does not occur, such as the contractions that occur when we press or pull against immovable objects. Although there has been some disagreement over the best way to improve strength and endurance, most authorities agree that resistance exercises involving movement (isotonic exercises) tend to produce the best results.

Recently, *isokinetics* has emerged as a type of strength-developing program. Isokinetic exercise combines all the advantages of isometrics and isotonics. This program makes use of specialized apparatus to provide a maximal resistance to the muscles (as in isometric exercises) but throughout their full range of movement (as in isotonics). Because of the need for expensive equipment, isokinetic training programs are not feasible for the average person. However, more and more fitness centers are providing such equipment for its members.

The Overload Principle

A muscle must be overloaded to be strengthened. The development of strength results from an increase in the thickness of the muscle fibers within a muscle rather than from an increase in their number. The increase in fiber size is called *hypertrophy.* Hypertrophy and the corresponding improvements in strength are produced by giving a muscle a greater-than-normal load.

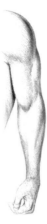

Systematic and progressive overloading of a muscle increases its strength. Generally, the degree of improvement is directly related to the degree of overload. Once a muscle has adapted to a higher demand, an additional increase in the load is necessary to produce further gains. In progressive-resistance exercises (such as training with barbells and weights) a muscle is made to contract against a resistance that requires a maximal or near-maximal contraction.

As a general rule lifting against a heavy load (more weight and few repetitions) tends to build maximum strength and muscle size. Lifting a lighter poundage with more repetitions tends to build muscular endurance along with good muscular definition and tone. For the average adult we strongly recommend the latter approach for developing strength and endurance.

The Effects of Muscular Development in Women

The beneficial effects of progressive-resistance exercise programs have been demonstrated for both men and women. Women normally have less muscle mass than men. However, there is as much variance among women in muscle mass development as there is among men. Thus, some women are stronger than some men.

Many women fear that exercising with barbells and weights will make them overly muscular and unfeminine-looking. There is no scientific basis to this fear. The inherent capacity for muscle development is genetically determined by sex hormone levels. The male hormone, testosterone, causes the muscle bulkiness in males. Even though this hormone is present in women, the amount is too low to have a substantial effect on muscle size. Dr. Jack Wilmore, an exercise physiologist, has compared the increase in strength of college-age men and women after a ten-week weight-training program. The women made substantial gains in strength, as did the men. When leg strength was expressed relative to body weight, the values for women and men were almost identical. However, the men's muscle size increased almost twice as much as the women's. Doctor Wilmore's findings support the theory that women can increase their strength significantly without a corresponding increase in muscle bulk. Therefore, weight training in women seems to produce a trim, well-contoured figure, rather than bulky, masculine muscles.

Utilizing the Basic Twelve

In Chapter 7, we laid out a series of exercises (the Basic Tweleve) that is primarily aimed at stretching the muscles for flexibility. The Basic Twelve can also be used for muscular development. Increasing the number of repetitions (application of the overload principle) for each exercise can help you improve your strength and muscular endurance.

In addition to the Basic Twelve, we strongly suggest adding two exercises to your program: sit-ups to strengthen your abdominal muscles, and push-ups to strengthen the muscles in your upper body region (arms, shoulders, chest).

Bent-Knee Sit-Ups

The sit-up exercise is a must in every muscular strength and endurance program. The abdominal muscles are difficult to involve in our everyday activities. However, these muscles are important in supporting the back and the various upper structures of our body. They also play a prominent role in maintaining our posture and holding in our stomachs.

Procedure: (See Figure 26.) Lie on your back with your feet under a couch or a firm support (a friend may hold your feet). It helps if you can find a soft surface, like a carpet, to lie on. Bend your knees approximately 90°. Put your feet flat on the floor, and interlock your hands behind your neck, elbows folded forward toward your knees. Now curl your back and raise your trunk until it's perpendicular to the floor. Then, return to the starting position on the floor. It is very important that your knees are flexed throughout the exercise. Doing sit-ups with your legs straight tends to strengthen your big hip-flexors, not your abdominal muscles. When the knees are bent, these large muscles are

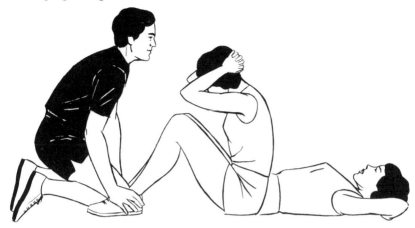

Figure 26. Bent-knee sit-ups.

less apt to be involved and the strength and endurance of your abdominal muscles provide the force to raise your trunk from the floor. The curling action of your trunk also provides a good strengthening and stretching stimulus to the lower back muscles.

Sit-Backs (A Modified Approach)

People beginning our program are often unable to do even one sit-up. Don't be alarmed if you fall into this category. The following procedure will show you how you can improve the strength of your abdominal muscles so that you can do sit-ups.

Procedure: First, sit on the floor with your knees flexed and feet under a couch or firm support as in Figure 26. In an upright sitting position place your hands behind the head with fingers interlaced and back rounded (curled). Now slowly lower your upper body to the floor. When you get almost half-way back, hold the position, keeping the back curled (the hands interlaced behind the neck helps). Keep the back curled to ease unnecessary strain on front neck muscles. Most likely you will begin to feel a vibration in the muscles of your abdominal region. Hold this position for a few moments, trying to bear some of the discomfort. Then let your upper body go all the way back to the floor and rest there for a moment. Now, using your elbows and hands, raise your upper body back into a sitting position and repeat this exercise a few times. Each day, increase the number of repeats until you can do ten in one workout. Then on the next day, test yourself by starting in the position with your back on the floor, hands interlaced behind your neck, and see if you can raise your head and shoulders to your knees in a curled position. If you can, lower yourself back to the floor and try to do another. If you can do one or two — great! This is progresss, and with time your muscles will get stronger and you will eventually be able to do 20 or more sit-ups a day — a reasonable goal.

You must be careful not to pull a muscle by overdoing it, so don't be in a hurry. If you do bent-knee sit-ups on a regular basis, be sure to do other exercises that stretch the hip flexors. The reason for this is that during the sit-up, the abdominal muscles are only involved for the first part of the curling up movement. Such exercises as the alternate arm and leg lifter and the quad stretcher (see the Basic Twelve) will help offset the overdevelopment of the hip flexors.

If you can already do 10 to 15 sit-ups, we encourage you to maintain this and try to increase the repetitions to 20 to 30 at a time. It is not uncommon for men and women, regardless of age, to be able to do 50 to 60 sit-ups during a two-minute period. However, 20 to 30 sit-ups per day in 60 seconds is usually sufficient for maintaining reasonable tone of the abdominal muscles.

Push-Ups

Push-ups will improve the strength in the upper body region. As with sit-ups, many men and women who start in our program can't do even one push-up. If you cannot do push-ups, don't despair. We will show you how. Follow the procedure below:

Procedure: Stand with feet together facing a wall about an arm's length away. Put your hands against the wall at shoulder height. Lean forward until your chest comes near the wall and push back to the starting position, as illustrated in Figure 27a. Try to repeat the exercise ten times or until the effort becomes too tough. If you can do ten repetitions after a brief rest try to repeat another set of ten. The next day when you work out, try to do ten push-aways again. As this exercise becomes easier, increase the number of push-aways until you can do two complete sets of 10 to 15. Once you can do two sets, then shift your position by moving further from the wall so that your hands are lower on the wall and you are in a more horizontal position.(See Figure 27b.) Keep striving to complete two sets of 10 to 15 each day while your hands move lower on the wall. If you find these too easy, then try a stairway or a counter in a kitchen or bathroom. When you find a position where completing ten push-aways is somewhat tough, then you have found

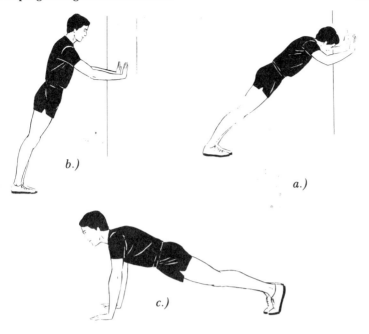

Figure 27a, b, and c. Push-ups.

your starting point. Eventually you can put your hands on the floor with your toes in a full push-up position, as illustrated in Figure 27c.

By now you realize that as the push-aways become easier, you increase the resistance to your upper arm and shoulder muscles by putting your body in a position that allows for a greater weight to be moved. The purpose of this is to increase your strength so you can handle your body weight at least ten times in a full push-up position. We feel this is a reasonable goal for attaining a minimal amount of upper body strength for both men and women

Additional Exercises for Walkers and Runners

Walking and running on a regular basis can have some bad effects on the muscles of the legs. We have stressed the importance of stretching the muscles in the back of your legs before and after each workout. As you increase the time and distance of your workouts, your large running-walking muscles on the back of your thighs and calves become very tight. In addition, these same muscles become stronger, which can lead to strength imbalances, causing injuries. Therefore, you need to strengthen the opposing muscles on the front of your legs.

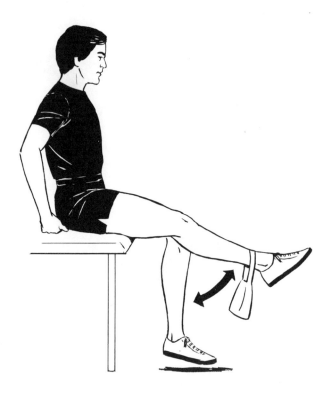

Figure 28. Quadricep strengthener

Quadricep strengthener. The quadricep strengthener (Figure 28) strengthens the front muscles of the thigh (quadriceps), which are the main extensors of the knee. This exercise helps to offset the increased strength and endurance development of the rear thigh muscles (hamstrings).

Procedure: Sit on a table with legs hanging down. Put a five- to ten-pound weight over the toes. (A handbag weighted down with canned goods should do). Holding on to the sides of the table, straighten (extend) the leg at the knee. Hold for a moment and return to the starting position. Relax, then repeat for one to two minutes. Then do the same for the other leg.

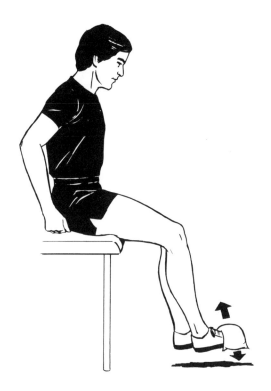

Figure 29. Lower leg strengthener.

Lower-leg flexor. The lower-leg flexor (Figure 29) serves to strengthen the muscles on front of the lower leg (often called dorsiflexor muscles). These muscles are often very weak in inactive people.

Procedure: Sit on a table with legs hanging down. This time, put only a two- to four-pound weight over your toes. Flex your foot at the ankle by drawing your toes up toward your knee. Return to the starting position. Repeat for one to 2-minutes by flexing up slowly and lowering the toes slowly. Then do the same for the other leg.

Up to now we have provided a few simple exercises for strength and muscular development. These exercises were not recommended to build large bulky muscles, but to build muscles that can help you to be reasonably effective in your everyday living. In fact, I feel that regular attention to the Basic Twelve, sit-ups, push-ups, and the quadricep and lower leg strengtheners are all you need to complement adequately your cardiorespiratory exercise program (walking, running, cycling, or swimming).

Training With Weights

I'm sure that by now you are fully aware that the training of your cardiorespiratory system should receive most of your emphasis. Nevertheless, many adults enjoy the challenge of strength development, especially if proper equipment for overloading muscles is readily available. To serve this interest, I will now offer some basic recommendations for a personalized weight-training program.

A weight-training program should systematically impose demands on muscle groups of the body. These imposed demands (such as barbell resistance) must be individualized and gradually intensified if you are to develop your maximal strength capabilities. Although weight training is a vigorous activity, it does not significantly improve cardiorespiratory endurance. However, it can be an important supplement to your program for developing circulatory and respiratory function.

Basic Equipment

The beginning program presented here requires the use of a barbell and disks of various weights. This equipment can be purchased at most sporting goods stores, and all the exercises can be done at home. If you belong to a fitness center, health club, or YW / YMCA, most likely you have weights readily available there. Many such facilities also have such sophisticated equipment as Nautilus machines, the Universal Gym, Total Gym, and other strength-development equipment. If you normally do your running or swimming at these sites, it will be easy to incorporate a set routine of weight-resistance exercises to complement your rhythmic endurance-type training. The following guidelines can be easily adapted to the various weight machines, pulleys, and other specialized equipment. All the same, having your own barbell and weights at home may be more desirable and possibly less expensive.

The barbell is a steel bar five to six feet long with a collar for holding the weighted disks in place at each end of the bar. Standard sets usually contain disks of $2\frac{1}{2}$, 5, 10, and 25 pounds. Normally, the barbell and collars together weigh around 25 pounds. The number of weighted disks required depends on the type of program. For the program we recommend, a man would need about 175 pounds of weights for the bar. For a woman, 125 pounds would suffice.

Weight-Training Terms

For understanding the procedures and techniques of weight-training, it helps if you are familiar with some basic terminology. The term *repetitions* refers to the number of contractions per bout, or set. For instance, if you curl a barbell ten consecutive times, you have completed one set of ten repetitions (reps). The total poundage (bar, disks, and collars) used for the exercise is referred to as the *load*. The maximum load that can be lifted a given number of times is called the *repetitions maximum* (RM). Therefore, the "Ten RM" means the greatest weight that can be lifted ten times for a given exercise. Likewise, "15 RM" refers to the maximum load that can be lifted 15 times for a given exercise.

Safety Precautions

The quality of your weight-training program depends largely on the proper performance of the selected exercises. Improper techniques of lifting can result in injury. Working out with the assistance of a partner, or spotter, is recommended.

When lifting the barbell and weights from the floor to begin an exercise, make sure you lift with the legs and not with the lower back. You do this by placing your feet close to the bar, lowering your hips to a squat position, head up and back straight. Then lift by straightening the legs. Always check to see that the barbell collars are tight and properly fastened on the bar to prevent the weights from falling off. Also, when you are lifting a heavy weight load (especially during the bench press, heel lifts, and half squats), be sure you have spotters (helpers) to assist you in getting the barbell into position and to remove it when you have completed your set of repetitions. Wear gymwear, especially rubber-soled footware to ensure stability during each exercise. In addition, make sure you follow a proper progression for adjusting the weight load. Too heavy a load at the start can cause unnecessary injury. You should finish your workout comfortably tired, not exhausted.

Principles and Procedures

An abundance of research has dealt with the most effective ways to train with weights. The recommended principles and procedures that follow are based on conclusions from such recent research.

Weight training programs that range from two RM for one set to ten RM for three sets all produce signifigant strength gain. Dr. Richard Berger, a Temple University researcher in muscular strength and endurance, asserts that the optimal training combination is Six RM for three sets, three times a week. My own experiences with weight-training programs for young adult men and women support Dr. Berger's conclusions. I feel confident in recommending a regimen of six RM, three sets, three times a week for young people. However, for the average adult such effort could be dangerous. The very nature of the exercise — short bursts of exertion against a heavy resistance — creates large increases in blood pressure, causing a heavy strain on the heart. Therefore, if you are beginning a strength-development program, I suggest a milder approach: lighter barbell loads with more repetitions; *e.g., 15-20 RM for three sets, three times a week.*

The following exercises comprise only a beginning program for men and women. The recommended training workout takes about 20 minutes of actual lifting. However, the availability of equipment and the time involved in changing the weight loads can lengthen the duration of your workout.

As you begin your weight-training program, use the barbell without the weighted disks. Learn the correct movements of the various exercises first, then proceed to add barbell disks (weights) for added resistance.

For optimum results, keep an accurate record of each workout on a chart like the one shown in the following table. Record the load and reps for each exercise. These records will help you regulate your workouts accurately. Remember to increase the load after you can easily complete three sets of 15 to 20 repetitions for a certain load. In addition, avoid doing the same exercises consecutively. If possible, do one set of curls, then bent-over rowing, then return to do your second set of curls. Such a pattern minimizes some of the muscular fatigue associated with weight-training. However, if you have access to only one set of weights, then in terms of the time spent it is best to complete all three sets before changing the weighted disks for the next exercise. There is no need to follow a particular sequence.

A warm-up period of conditioning exercises that involve stretching should precede your weight-training routine. These are needed to loosen the muscles and stimulate the circulation. The Basic Twelve will do. (Refer to Chapter 7, if needed.)

Your beginning load for each exercise can be determined by trial

EXERCISE		10/4	10/6	10/8	10/11	10/13	10/15	10/18			
CURL	LB	25	25	25	35	35					
	RM	15-14-12	15-14-14	15-15-15	12-10-9	12-11-9					
PRESS	LB	35	35	35	35	35					
	RM	12-10-10	12-12-10	14-12-15	15-13-12	15-15-13					
BENCH PRESS	LB	40	40	50	50	50					
	RM	15-15-13	15-15-15	12-10-8	12-10-10	14-10-10					
UPRIGHT ROWING	LB	40	50	50	50	50					
	RM	15-15-15	15-10-10	15-10-10	15-12-10	15-14-12					
BENT-OVER ROWING	LB	50	50	60	60	60					
	RM	15-15-12	15-15-15	10-10-6	12-10-8	12-12-8					
HEEL LIFTS	LB	70	70	70	70	70					
	RM	12-10-10	12-12-10	12-12-10	14-12-10	15-13-10					
HALF SQUATS	LB	70	70	70	70	70					
	RM	15-15-12	15-15-15	15-10-10	15-12-10	15-15-12					

and error. An easy way to approximate it is based on your body weight. Your body weight corresponds roughly to your strength. Therefore, each exercise description suggests the portion of your body weight for a beginning load. When you can easily perform more than 15 to 20 reps (on the third set) for a given exercise, then add five to ten pounds or more at your next training session. By following these procedures for three sessions a week, you will experience significant gains in six to eight weeks.

Remember, your goal is not muscle bulk but reasonable improvement in strength, muscular endurance, and muscle definition (tone). As you get your cardiorespiratory system in better shape (from walking, running, swimming, or cycling), it may be safe for you to lift heavier weights with fewer repetitions. But for most of us, the resulting additional strength isn't necessary in order to function in today's society.

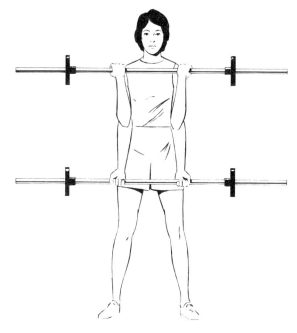

Figure 30. Arm curls.

ARM CURLS

Purpose:	To develop the flexors of the arms and forearms.
Starting Position:	Stand erect, arms fully extended downward, and hold the barbell with an underhand grip (palms outward); your hands should be shoulder-width apart.
Movement:	Raise the barbell to your chest by flexing your arms. Your elbows should remain at your sides. Then, lower to the starting position. If possible, stand erect with your back to a wall.
Suggested Beginning Load:	One-eighth to one-fourth of your body weight.

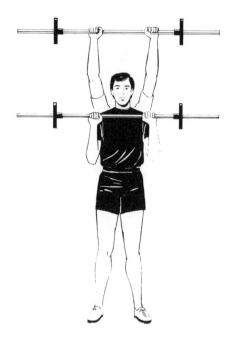

Figure 31. The press.

PRESS

Purpose:	To develop the extensors of the upper arms and the muscles of the shoulder, back, and upper chest region.
Starting Position:	Stand erect. Grasp the barbell with your thumbs pointing inward (overhand grip) and in a resting position on your upper chest with elbows down.
Movement:	Push (raise) the bars straight overhead until your arms lock. Then lower the bar back to chest position.
Suggested Beginning Load:	One-eighth to one-fourth of your body weight.

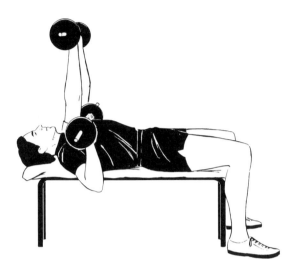

Figure 32. Benchpress.

BENCH PRESS*

Purpose:	To develop muscles of the chest and shoulders and the extensors of the arm (triceps).
Starting Position:	Lie on your back on a bench with your knees bent and your feet flat on the floor, straddling the bench. Have a friend hand you the barbell in a position above your chest, with arms up and elbows locked. Your hands should be placed slightly wider than the breadth of your shoulders, thumbs under and palms upward.
Movement:	Lower the barbell to middle of chest and then press it back to the extended position.
Suggested Beginning Load:	One-fourth to one-third of your body weight.

*Spotters at each end of the barbell are recommended for this exercise.

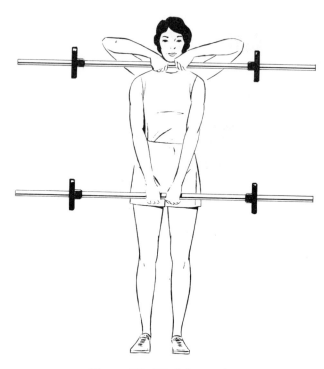

Figure 33. Upright rowing.

UPRIGHT ROWING

Purpose: To develop the shoulder, back, and arm muscles.

Starting Position: Stand erect, arms down, hold the barbell across your thighs with an overhand grip (thumbs in), hands one to three inches apart.

Movement: Raise the bar to a position at shoulder level under your chin. Keep your elbows above the bar throughout the exercise. Return to the starting position.

Suggested Beginning Load: One-fourth to one-third of your body weight.

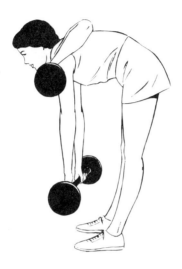

Figure 34. Bent-over rowing.

BENT-OVER ROWING

Purpose:	To develop the muscles of the back, back of shoulders, and front of upper arms.
Starting Position:	Bend at the waist with your upper body; your back is parallel to the floor. Extend your arms downward and grip the barbell with an overhand grip, hands shoulder-width apart.
Movement:	Bring the bar directly up to your chest, keeping your back straight and head up. Then return the bar to the extended position (a few inches off of the floor).
Suggested Beginning Load:	One-fourth to one-third of your body weight.

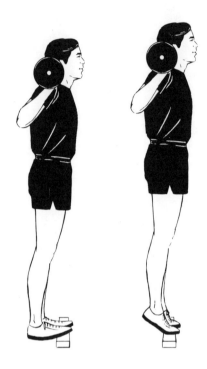

Figure 35. Heel lifts.

HEEL LIFTS*

Purpose:	To develop the muscles of the calves and feet.
Starting Position:	Stand erect with the barbell across your shoulders at the back of your neck. You may use padding on your back.
Movement:	Raise yourself on your toes to a fully extended position (heels off the floor) and then lower your heels slowly back to the floor. You can get an added range of motion by placing the balls of your feet over a stable two-by-four piece of wood.
Suggested Beginning Load:	One-third to one-half of your body weight.

*Spotters at each end of the barbell are recommended for this exercise.

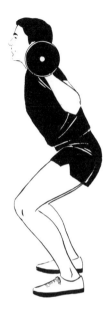

Figure 36. Half squats.

HALF-SQUATS*

Purpose:	To develop primarily the muscles of the upper legs.
Starting Position:	Stand erect with your feet shoulder-width apart, the barbell resting on your neck as for the heel lifts.
Movement:	Lower your body to a semi-squatting position by bending at the knees. Keep the back straight. Then return to a straight-knee position.
Suggested Beginning Load:	One-third to one-half of your body weight.

*Spotters at each end of the barbell are recommended for this exercise.

Summary

The basic exercises presented in this chapter provide a more than adequate program for firming up muscles, increasing muscle tone, and improving body contour and appearance. But, that's all!

According to claims by many strength enthusiasts, exercise workouts involving only weights (resistance) are all that is needed for developing total fitness. Unfortunately, scientific facts do not support these claims. It is common knowledge today based on expert research that strength training does not stress the heart and lungs adequately for improving the strength and efficiency of the cardiorespiratory system. Recall that throughout this book we have emphasized the importance of engaging big muscles in vigorous and rhythmic movements over an extended period of time. Such activities (e.g., running, swimming, cycling) expend large amounts of energy (calories). Since the muscles need large amounts of oxygen to produce ample quantities of energy (ATP) to perform rhythmic endurance-type activities, the development of the cardiorespiratory system to deliver the oxygen to the muscle cells is important. Scientific studies clearly show that weight training or any similar resistance-type training doesn't stimulate the energy systems (oxygen uptake) and the heart adequately to bring about significiant physiological change.

You must engage your large muscle masses in sustained vigorous exercise to achieve a cardiorespiratory training effect. As I have emphasized throughout this book, this simply means regular participation (at least four times a week, 30 minutes a day) in an activity that raises and sustains your heart beat at a 75% heart rate reserve level. Strength and muscular endurance training, although a big muscle activity, doesn't require a high level of energy expenditure. Nevertheless, a program aimed at improving your strength and muscular endurance may be important to your needs. I hope, however, that your cardiorespiratory fitness program is not neglected or excluded in favor of a strength-training program. Having strength and muscular endurance is important but not at the expense of neglecting your cardiorespiratory training.

chapter fourteen

Nutrition, Weight Control, and Exercise

Being physically fit involves keeping our weight under control. Keeping off excess body fat is a continual struggle for most of us. This chapter presents the suggestions and guidelines used in our program at Ball State for those who have weight problems and want help with this aspect of being fit.

Food has always been at the center of our lives. Eating, although a necessity, is often viewed as a recreation — something we do in leisure-time for pleasure. In a recent Harris survey, 84% of Americans named eating as their top leisure-time activity. We snack in front of the TV and at athletic events; we go out to eat at our favorite restaurants. Preparation of hearty and tasty meals is a way of showing affection for others; holiday feasts, cocktail parties, and backyard barbeques are part of our social routine. Business transactions are frequently conducted over food and drink. Unfortunately all this enjoyable abandon can lead to excess poundage or even outright obesity.

Obesity (excessive fat) is a major public health problem. It affects over 50% of the American adult population. It's the most prevalent form of malnutrition in the United States and studies indicate that it's increasing.

Obesity has far-reaching complications. It's closely related to cardiovascular, respiratory, kidney, and gall bladder diseases, as well as to diabetes, disorders of bones and joints, and, in some, emotional imbalance. Obese persons are more prone to fatigue (increasing the risk of accidents), indigestion, and constipation, and have numerous aches and pains. Besides having to cope with the psychological effects of being fat, they face premature death.

Most people who are fat don't want to be, so the fight against fat rages on. Our newstands and bookstores are deluged with publications

265

dealing with nutrition and weight control. Over the past few years, cookbooks and books on dieting have been at the top of the bestseller charts. Reducing salons and weight-watching clubs abound.

The American public spends over $10 billion each year trying to win the battle of the bulge. At the same time, the food industry invests millions of dollars to develop and offer new products and items for the fast-food market. On the other hand, advertisements frequently promote the fast or easy way to get rid of excess fat. We constantly worry about what to eat and how to get rid of what we've already eaten.

Today, one of the key issues in weight control is the ineffectiveness of current treatments. Only about one-fourth of the patients are successful in losing weight, and many regain it after treatment ends. Statistics show that 50% of those who go on a diet quit after one year, 70% after two years. According to the American Medical Association, only 5% are truly successful — taking off excess fat and keeping it off.

In order to treat obesity effectively, we have to deal with its causes. We have a proclivity for food, and in most of America, food is plentiful. Social factors encourage over-consumption. The truth is, though, that *excess body fat is caused not so much by increased consumption as by decreased activity.*

If you are overweight, most likely you've tried all kinds of diets and exercise programs but have little or nothing to show for all your effort. You've lost money and time. You don't need to invest your money in fancy gadgets to lose weight and keep it off, but you *do* need to invest your time and effort. No one can do it for you and you can't buy slimness. With proper knowledge of some specific weight control skills, one being proper exercise, you can begin to effectively learn how to achieve a lifetime program for weight control.

The Basic Principle of Weight Control

The basic principle of weight control is simple. Your energy intake (food) and your energy output (physical activity) must be kept in balance. When you eat more than you need for daily energy, the excess energy is stored as body fat. When you eat less the stored fat is burned for energy. Grasping this principle isn't hard, but putting it into practice is.

It's obvious from this basic principle that we must not only watch what we eat but what we do. Going on a strict diet won't be effective in the long run unless we get active. Regular exercise coupled with sound eating habits offer the most sensible approach to controlling weight.

Controlling weight must be a lifetime activity. We often say we're "going on" a diet. This implies that someday we're "coming off" that diet. Going on and off diets is not the way to manage our body weight. If losing weight is necessary, then the loss must be gradual (no more than two pounds per week).

Nutrition Basics

Nutrition is the study of the food we eat and how the body uses it. A sound understanding of the basics of nutrition is important in our lifetime commitment to weight control.

Food provides a wide variety of necessary substances, or nutrients. These substances are essential for building and repairing the body, and for energy. There are three basic classes of nutrients in the food we eat: proteins, carbohydrates, and fats. Minerals, vitamins, and water are also essential for life but do not provide energy. Here is a brief summary of the role of each nutrient.

Protein

Protein is the basic structural substance of each cell in the body. It provides structure to bones, skin, muscle fibers, and many tissues. It is the basic material of enzymes and hormones that control and regulate chemical reactions in our bodies. Specialized proteins present in blood serve as clotting agents and oxygen-carrying molecules. When we eat, proteins in food are broken down into amino acids. These amino acids travel through the bloodstream and are then combined in various parts of the body to form the structures just mentioned (various kinds of cells).

The major sources of protein are foods of animal origin: meat, fish, poultry, eggs, milk. Nutritionists also suggest peas, beans, and nuts as good substitutes for animal protein. About 15% of the calories we consume each day should come from protein.

Carbohydrates

Carbohydrates (starches and sugars) provide energy; that is, fuel for performing bodily functions, such as forming new chemical compounds, transmitting nerve impulses, and supplying the primary energy for muscular activity. (In contrast, proteins are not used significantly for energy during physical activity.) Good sources of starches are potatoes, beans, peas, grains (wheat, oats, corn, and rice), flour, macaroni, spaghetti, noodles, grits, bread, cakes, and breakfast cereal. Sweets such as candy, jams, jellies, table sugar, honey, molasses, and concentrated syrups provide sugars. Fruits, vegetables, and fruit juices also contain carbohydrates.

Currently there is much confusion about eating sugar, a carbohydrate, and its possible adverse affects on the body. Doesn't the body need sugar? Yes, but our bodies do not need all the extra sugar added to foods. (Sugar, as used in this chapter, refers to *sucrose* or refined sugar, whereas blood sugar — the end product of carbohydrate breakdown — refers to *glucose*.)

There are many other forms of carbohydrates: lactose — a sugar found in milk; fructose — a fruit sugar; and starches. All of these forms of carbohydrates serve the same basic purpose: to provide glucose for the body. The key point, however, is that the foods that contain milk sugar, fruit sugar, and starches also supply other needed nutrients; they do more than satisfy our sweet tooth. They provide many of the minerals and vitamins essential for an adequate diet. But refined sugar doesn't.

Many nutritionists feel overeating refined sugar (the stuff you put in coffee and on your cereal), especially the sugars found in many processed foods, is largely responsible for several dangerous diseases. Obesity, heart disease, and adult-onset diabetes have been linked to overeating sugar. Also, it is well established that tooth decay is related to eating sugar-based foods.

Sugar must be consumed in moderation and not to the exclusion of other important foods in your diet. The problem with sugar-based foods is that they taste so good that the average American consumes well over 100 pounds of refined sugar per year. Much of this sugar is hidden in the processed foods that we eat regularly. These are called *empty calorie* foods because they provide nothing but energy. It seems wise to cut down on sugar intake by avoiding sweet snacks and foods high in sugar. In other words, select foods that provide a good nutrient return for the caloric investment.

The overeating of sugars may rob our bodies of the necessary vitamins and minerals that result from a well-balanced diet. The more refined sugar you can eliminate from your daily eating, the better. Nutritionist Dr. Jean Mayer sums it up well: "About the only good thing I can say for sugar is that it tastes good!"

Approximately 55% of the calories you consume each day should come from carbohydrates, and 40% of that should be carbohydrates other than refined sugar. This means eating more vegetables, fruits, and starches. Whenever you take in more carbohydrates than your body needs, the excess is converted to fat and stored. Hence, a person who eats too many calories of carbohydrates is sure to increase the body's fat content.

Fats

The main components of fats — fatty acids — are a concentrated source of energy and provide more than twice as much energy (calories) as comparable amounts of either carbohydrates or protein. Fat is a necessary nutrient. Besides being an important part of the cell structure, fat acts as an insulator and protector of vital parts of the body, and provides additional energy for muscular activity. Common sources of fats are fatty meats (bacon, hamburger), butter, margarine, shortening, cooking and salad oils, cream, most cheeses, mayonnaise, nuts, milk, eggs, and chocolate. Of course, anything cooked in fat contains fat.

There are two basic types of fats: saturated and unsaturated. Saturated fats come from meat, whole milk, cheese, and butter (that is, from animals). This type of fat does not melt at room temperature. In contrast, unsaturated fats come from vegetables and tend to be liquid at room temperature. Saturated fats raise levels of cholesterol in the bloodstream. Because of this, many nutritionists and physicians are trying to persuade people to reduce the saturated fats in their diet. Approximately 30% of the calories you consume each day should come from fats, more from unsaturated than saturated fats. Unsaturated fats (liquid fats) are found in peanut and olive oils. Polyunsaturated (more liquid) fats are found in corn, soybean, cottonseed, and particularly, safflower oils. It is believed that if you reduce your intake of solid fats to a minimum and use unsaturated or polyunsaturated fats as an alternative to animal fat, you will lower the levels of serum cholesterol.

Cholesterol, a fat-like substance, is found only in animal products, especially egg yolks, liver, brain, shrimp, lobster, and other crustacean

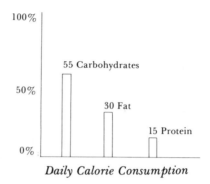

Daily Calorie Consumption

foods. Cholesterol is necessary in the body, and your body can produce some of what it needs. It is required for many of the complex functions of the body and is used in making the important sex hormones. When there is too much of it, however, it tends to settle in the walls of the blood vessels and can impair circulation.

Minerals

The body requires many minerals. They give strength and rigidity to certain body tissues and assist with numerous vital functions. Calcium, iodine, iron, phosphorous, magnesium, and others are vitally important to the functioning of body systems. Calcium is the most abundant mineral in the body and combines with phosphorous to form the teeth and bones. Calcium is also crucial for the normal functioning of muscles. Phosphorus is an essential component for supplying energy to the body. Iodine is an important ingredient to thyroxin, a hormone that governs the rate of energy metabolism in the body. Iron is a key component of hemoglobin in the blood.

Sodium and potassium play a key role in controlling and regulating fluid balance in the body. These elements, called electrolytes, are mainly present in the fluids inside and surrounding the cells and are essential for proper transmission of nerve impulses. Sodium is present in all living matter, such as meats, poultry, fish, and vegetables. It is added in the processing of food as a preservative and stabilizer and is used as table salt to flavor food. It is well known that the sodium we consume contributes to high blood pressure. Medical doctors strongly recommend limiting our sodium intake by not salting food and avoiding products containing sodium additives. A recent decision by baby-food processors to discontinue adding salt to their products demonstrates national awareness of the dangers of excess salt in the diet. As a general rule, balanced meals supply all the minerals you need.

Vitamins

Vitamins are organic substances that the body needs in small amounts for the proper functioning of muscles and nerves. They also play a dynamic role in releasing energy from foods and in promoting normal growth of body tissues. The cells of the body cannot form these substances, and therefore the vitamins needed by the body must be provided by the food you eat.

Some vitamins tend to be retained within the body, stored in fat. Other vitamins are transported in the fluids of the tissues and cells and are not stored. The latter vitamins must be consumed in the daily diet and any excessive intake is usually excreted in the urine. Therefore, ingesting more vitamins than recommended will be of limited or no benefit. In fact, excessive intake of vitamins can be harmful. Medical research has documented the toxicity of large doses of vitamin intake. All the required vitamins can be found in well-rounded nutritious diet. Healthy people who eat well-balanced meals do not need vitamin supplements.

Water

The body's need for water exceeds its need for food. About three-fourths of your body is water, and water is second only to oxygen in importance. Water provides the medium (body fluids) for transporting nutrients and hormones throughout the body and for removing wastes from the body. Water also plays a vital role in regulating body temperature. You get the water you need not only by drinking it directly but from the foods you eat.

National Dietary Goals

The growing recognition of the importance of nutrition in weight control and health has led to a need for basic goals and practical guides for an individual to follow. A Senate Committee on Nutrition and Human Needs published a report in 1977 focusing on the health concerns related to the eating patterns of the average American. This report generated widespread interest and controversy. It stated that the composition of our diet has changed radically in recent years. The complex carbohydrates (from fruit, vegetables, and grain), previously the mainstay of the diet, have now been replaced by increased consumption of fat and refined sugars. These changes are considered detrimental to our health. This overconsumption of fat and sugar, along with increased intake of cholesterol, salt, and alcohol, has been related to six of the ten leading causes of death in the United States. In an attempt to combat this health problem, the committee recommended six dietary goals that represent "prudent" eating habits and seven guidelines for changes in food selection and preparation. The guidelines are as follows:

1. To avoid being overweight, consume only as much energy (calories) as is expended; if overweight, decrease energy intake and increase energy expenditure.
2. Increase the eating of complex carbohydrates (naturally occuring sugars and starches) such as fruits, vegetables, and grains.
3. Decrease the consumption of refined and processed sugars to 15% of your total energy intake.
4. Reduce the overall consumption of fat to about 30% of your energy intake.
5. Reduce saturated fat consumption to 10% and balance that with polyunsaturated fats.
6. Reduce cholesterol consumption to about 300 milligrams a day.
7. Limit the intake of sodium by reducing the amount of salt consumed to about five grams a day.

If we accept these guidelines, the following adjustments in food selection and preparation must be made in our daily eating habits:

1. Eat less refined and other processed sugars and foods containing large amounts of such sugars.
2. Eat less foods high in animal fat and replace them with fats obtained from vegetable sources (polyunsaturated) or by choosing meats, poultry, and fish with low amounts of saturated fat.
3. Eat less butterfat, eggs, and other dairy products that are high in cholesterol. Substitute low-fat and non-milk for whole milk.
4. Eat less salt and foods high in salt content.
5. Eat more fruits, vegetables, and whole grain products.

It is important to note that the committee recognizes that these dietary recommendations do not guarantee protection from the killer diseases; they do, however, increase the probability of improved protection. These guidelines have been suggested to assist you in making wise food choices that are consistent with good health. The combination of sound nutritional habits and regular vigorous activity can enhance your health.

Caloric Values of Food

All the energy released from our food intake becomes heat in the body. This energy expenditure, as well as the potential energy in foods, is measured in calories.

Numerous books on diet and nutrition contain long lists of the calorie content of various foods. If you wish to formulate a weight-loss or a weight-maintenance diet, you will need such information to plan your daily diet. Since there are often discrepancies in the caloric values of food in diet books, it's best to use the *Nutritive Value of American Foods in Common Units* (Agricultural Handbook # 456, U.S. Department of Agriculture, Washington, D.C., 1975).

Overweight and Obesity

The energy, or caloric, needs of your body depend on factors such as your body size, age, and the type and amount of your daily physical activity. We all need the same nutrients, but in different amounts. Young people need greater quantities of food for body growth, upkeep, and energy. Large people need more food than small people. Construction workers need more food than office workers. However, no matter what your energy needs are, if you take in more calories than your daily activities use up, you gain weight.

Many people like to believe that an abnormality in their metabolism is the reason for their being overweight. Some insist it's inherited. Medical research does not support these theories. Gland malfunction is most likely not the reason for obesity. Fatness runs in families, but often it is a result of social or environmental factors rather than genetic factors. Most likely, our inactive way of life is the real culprit. We just don't burn off the calories we eat each day, and therefore, the surplus energy is stored in the fat cells of the body.

Recent research has indicated that human fat cells increase in number very rapidly in early life and, once formed, become fixed for life. When infants are overfed, they tend to produce more fat cells, which make weight control more difficult later in life. A fat baby is not necessarily a healthy baby. Preventive steps should be taken at an early age to curb this potential for unnecessarily multiplying an infant's fat cells.

Overfeeding in infancy is frequently followed by forced feeding in early childhood. Demanding children to clean their plates before leaving the table and using sweets to reward them cultivates habits that could haunt them as they grow older. Sound nutritional habits begin at home.

What's Your Ideal Weight

In determining your ideal weight, how much fat you have is more important than how much you weigh. Many people quickly turn to the standard height-weight tables (reflecting life insurance standards) for guidelines. These tables are derived from measurements of a great variety of people. Although they enable us to compare ourselves with the average man and woman, they are often inadequate guides to ideal weight. Many athletes who are low in body fat but very muscular could be overweight according to these charts. Also, some of these charts allow small increments in body weight with increasing age, a practice that lacks justification. Unmistakably, it is the proportion of fat tissue in your body, rather than your scale weight, that determines your proper weight.

In Chapter 5 we provide a means for estimating the percentage of body fat and for determining your desired weight. A body fat value between 10 and 12% of the total body weight is considered trim for adult men; by contrast, 18 to 20% body fat for women generally signifies trimness. More than 25% fat for men and over 30% for women indicate obesity—too much fat.

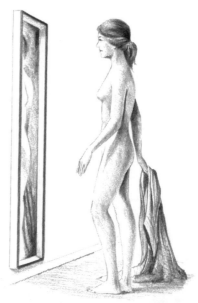

If you did not determine your percentage of fat by the method presented in Chapter 5 or the skinfold procedure in Appendix A, then an alternative is to look at your naked body in front of a full-length mirror. If you look fat, you are fat! Being able to pinch up about an inch of fat between your fingers in flabby areas of the body is a good indication that you have too much body fat. Remember, it is the proportion of fat tissue in the body's composition — rather than a reading on the bathroom scale — that determines if you are fat.

The Role of Exercise in Weight Control

Physical activity is the great variable in energy expenditure and can play a very important role in helping you control your body weight. Regular exercise and sound nutritional habits go hand in hand. You can lose weight just by dieting, but statistics show that you are less likely to regain weight if you combine a sound exercise program with your dieting.

Losing the Right Kind of Weight

You can always lose the wrong kind of weight. When weight is lost just from dieting, a significant amount of the weight loss comes from body water and lean (not fat) body tissue. Many people on a low-carbohydrate diet (depleting stored carbohydrate) experience quick weight loss due to the quick loss of body water. They are encouraged by the quick loss, yet deceived. Furthermore such crash diets will likely result in the loss of lean body tissue (from muscles, bones, and organs). When the crash diet ends and normal eating resumes, the weight regained will be mostly fat. It takes time to rebuild lean body tissues. When the weight is regained, the dieting often begins again, repeating the process. People who are constantly going on and off diets can jeopardize their health.

When a person starts an exercise program, a common occurrence is a gain in lean body weight associated with the build-up of muscle tissue. Even though there's a loss of body fat, total body weight changes little, since the build-up of lean tissue offsets the loss of body fat. This discourages some people since they do not see the needle drop on their bathroom scales. Don't be discouraged. The right kind of weight loss is occurring. After the body has adjusted to the regular exercise regimen, the build-up of muscle tissue levels off, but the burning off of stored fat continues. This loss *will* be reflected on the bathroom scale.

Determining Energy Expenditure

When exercise is used for weight reduction, the energy cost of physical activities should be considered in designing a weight-control program. It's necessary to determine your energy expenditure in order to balance it with your intake. Like potential energy in foods, the body's expenditure of energy is measured in calories. This energy expenditure is called the *caloric cost* of an activity. We can calculate the caloric costs by measuring the amount of heat given off by the body. Such measurement is extremely difficult during exercise. But since heat loss from energy expenditure is related to the amount of oxygen consumed by the body, rates of oxygen consumption can be used to measure energy expenditure.

One liter (approximately one quart) of oxygen consumed by the body during exercise is equivalent to approximately five calories of expended energy. When walking at 3.5 mph, a person of average size (150 lbs.) uses about five calories a minute, or 150 calories in 30 minutes. Since a 12-ounce can of beer contains about 150 calories, it would take 30 minutes of walking to burn off the calories consumed from the beer. Clearly, knowing the number of calories in food and the calories you spend in various physical activities can help you greatly in carrying out a sound weight-control program.

Energy Costs of Activities

In recent years, much research has been devoted to establishing the energy costs of various sports and exercises. When estimating energy expenditure for any individual, we must consider the time spent in the activity, the rate of work, and body size. The more time you spend at an activity, the more energy you use. Larger people tend to require more energy than smaller people for the same task. The tables on pages 278 and 280 show the energy cost expressed in calories per minute and in calories per minute per kilogram of body weight for walking, running, and selected sports. They will enable you to estimate your own caloric costs for selected activities.

These tables have been formulated from personal research and, in some cases, from research reported in professional journals. Activities that require five to nine calories/minute are considered moderate. Activities requiring above nine calories/minute are considered vigorous.

Each walking or running speed (page 278) is also expressed in terms of METs, another measure of caloric intensity. Remember, a MET refers to the rate of energy expended; one MET is equivalent to the energy needed at rest — approximately 1.25 calories a minute, or about a quarter of a liter of oxygen. Classifying an activity at seven METs, for instance, simply means that it requires seven times more energy than at a state of rest. Seven METs would be at the high end of moderate exercise; it is equivalent to 8.8 calories/minute, or a little more than 1.75 liters of oxygen uptake.

Anything over ten METs is considered vigorous. Marathon runners, who probably represent the zenith of cardiorespiratory fitness, run for two to three hours at an intensity level of 14 to 16 METs or more.

For estimating your energy cost for walking and running, first determine your kilogram body weight by multiplying your weight in pounds by .45 (1 pound equals .45 kilogram). Then select your preferred walking or running speed. Multiply your kilogram weight by the value under the column headed cal/min/kg in the energy table. This will be the caloric cost per minute for you.

For example, a 120-pound woman weighs 120 multiplied by .45 or 54 kg. Walking at a 17.5-minute-mile pace equals .0692, multiplied by 54 equals 3.7 calorie/minute. Running at a ten-minute-mile pace equals .1471, multiplied by 54 equals 7.9 calorie/minute. These rates equal 111 and 237 calories for 30 minutes of walking and running, respectively. A rate of 7.9 calories/minute would be classified as high-moderate whereas a rate of 3.7 calories/minute would be considered light. For a woman beginning a conditioning program, these may be adequate levels of intensity of exercise depending on her level of fitness. As always, the key determining factor is a person's own heart rate response.

If we take a 170-pound man (76.5 kg) running at an eight-minute-mile pace, he would require 14.2 calories/minute. This is a greater caloric cost than that of the woman just cited. He has a higher caloric cost because he is running at a faster tempo and carrying more body mass. Both factors require more energy. His heart rate response to this activity depends on his physical fitness. The better conditioned he is, the greater the caloric expenditure he can muster in a given period of time.

Let's compare two men, both weighing 68 kilograms. One can run four miles in 28 minutes (a seven-minute-mile pace) at a heart rate of 150 (an adequate training stimulus). The other can run 2.8 miles during the same time period (28 minutes at a ten-minute-mile pace) and at

ENERGY COST OF WALKING AND RUNNING

	CAL/MIN/KG	CAL/MIN				METS
		120-LB PERSON (54 KG)	150-LB PERSON (68 KG)	180-LB PERSON (81 KG)	200-LB PERSON (90 KG)	RANGE
20-min. mile (3 mph)	0.0577	3.1	3.9	4.6	5.2	2.5 to 4
17.5-min. mile (3.4 mph)	0.0692	3.7	4.7	5.6	6.2	3 to 5
15-min. mile (4 mph)	0.0872	4.7	5.9	7.1	7.8	4 to 6
10-min. mile (6 mph)	0.1471	7.9	10.0	11.9	13.2	6 to 11
8-min. mile (7.5 mph)	0.1856	10.0	12.6	15.0	16.7	8 to 13
7-min. mile (8 mph)	0.2118	11.4	14.4	17.2	19.1	9 to 15
6-min. mile (10 mph)	0.2350	12.7	16.0	19.0	21.2	10 to 17

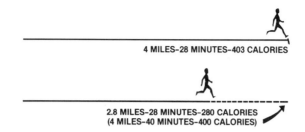

4 MILES–28 MINUTES–403 CALORIES

2.8 MILES–28 MINUTES–280 CALORIES
(4 MILES–40 MINUTES–400 CALORIES)

the same 150 heart rate. The first runner utilizes 403 calories for his workout; the second man can utilize only 280 calories during his workout. We can readily see that the man in better physical condition burns more calories during a 28-minute workout than the slower runner. This means more calories expended, a bonus for weight control. Now assume that the slower runner goes four miles, in other words, the same total distance as the 28-minute runner. He would then use another 120 calories, which would give him a similar caloric expenditure, 400 calories. But his total workout time is 40 minutes rather than 28. The runner who can run the four miles in 28 minutes has a greater functional fitness capacity than the slow runner. Nevertheless, for burning calories to control your weight, the most important factor is the distance you move, not the speed at which you move.

The following table presents caloric (energy) values for selected sports activities. The table is arranged in ascending order from the less intense activities (such as bowling) to a more intense activity — running a six-minute mile. Activities of below-moderate intensity, such as golf and bowling, do not represent a suitable means for developing or maintaining physical fitness. These sports, although considered to be aerobic activities, don't put enough stress on the cardiorespiratory system to produce a training effect. For weight control, however, activities such as golf can be beneficial. Although the cardiac and respiratory stimulus is minimal, extra calories are burned. If we again compare the 150-pound person who runs four miles in 28 minutes (a caloric cost of 403 calories), but this time with a golfer of the same weight, we find the golfer must play for a total of 106 minutes to burn the same 403 calories (106 multiplied by 3.8). Put another way, the golfer has to play (exercise) nearly four times as long as the runner for the same energy-cost benefits. Even worse, as we have seen, golf is not intense enough to produce a training effect on the heart and lungs, and thus is not suitable for developing cardiorespiratory fitness.

ENERGY COST OF SELECTED SPORTING ACTIVITIES

	CAL/MIN/KG	CAL/MIN*	METS*
Bowling (with three other bowlers)	0.0471	3.2	2.6
Golf (playing in a foursome)	0.0559	3.8	3.0
Walking (17.5-min. mile)	0.0692	4.7	3.8
Cycling (6.4-min. mile)	0.0985	6.7	5.4
Canoeing (15-min. mile)	0.1029	7.0	5.6
Swimming (59 yd/min.)	0.1333	9.1	7.3
Running (10-min. mile)	0.1471	10.0	8.0
Cycling (5-min. mile)	0.1559	10.6	8.5
Handball (singles)	0.1603	10.9	8.7
Rope skipping (80 turns/min.)	0.1655	11.3	9.0
Running (8-min. mile)	0.1856	12.6	10.1
Running (6-min. mile)	0.2350	16.0	12.8

*These are values for a 150-pound person (68 kg).

Some Common Misconceptions

Misconceptions about the relationship between exercise and weight control are quite common. Three of the most deceptive are: (1) exercise increases your appetite, (2) you can lose weight in spots, and (3) you can lose weight by just sweating.

Exercise and Appetite

Often we hear that if you exercise more, you will eat more. Dr. Jean Mayer, the renowned nutritionist, has concluded that a daily exercise session does not bring about a corresponding increase in appetite. Appetite is a fairly good guide to the amount of food needed by active people, but it is not a reliable measure for inactive people. Therefore, it does not follow that if you are inactive you will eat less than if you are active. Mayer's observations suggest that there is a range of inactivity in which the food intake no longer correlates with a decrease in activity. Thus, in that range there is an imbalance between food intake and energy output, and fatness results. Mayer calls this the "sedentary

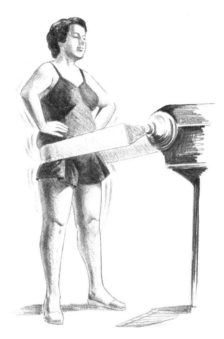

range." Above this range of inactivity is the range of normal activity, where appetite and exercise are attuned to each other.

Other studies have indicated that moderate to vigorous exercise of up to an hour in duration actually acts to depress the appetite. Although these studies are not conclusive, exercise seems to be a mild appetite suppressant, rather than an appetite stimulant.

Spot Reducing

Health spas and weight-reducing salons have often promoted programs for reducing. As consumers, you are frequently urged to use localized exercise or mechanical vibrators and other gadgets to reduce the fat in the flabby areas of your body. The evidence available today does not support the theory that if you exercise or massage a particular area of your body, you will reduce the excess fat in that region. Calisthenics, yoga, or "slimnastics" might be beneficial to general muscle tone and flexibility, but they do not reduce fat tissue in specific locations.

Regular exercise that is vigorous and continuous, involving total body movement, does reduce skinfold fat and girth measurements. When fat is reduced, it tends to be reduced all over the body, in proportion to the amount present at any given site. Muscles do not use just the fat stored near them. Whenever you use a muscle or a group of muscles, hormone signals go to the fat storage depots throughout your body. These cells release fat molecules into the blood-stream which takes them to the working muscle to be used as fuel. In other words, during vigorous exercise you draw from your total fat reserves. Activities that vigorously stress the cardiorespiratory system provide the best means for fat reduction.

Weight Reduction by Sweating

Many people purposely overheat their bodies, hoping for a quick loss of excess body weight. Exercising in hot, humid weather, or while wearing a rubber sweat suit, or even sitting in a steam room after exercise are common methods for prompting profuse sweating. Although your reading on the scales may be temporarily lower by a pound or two, this weight loss has nothing to do with body fat and will not be permanent.

Sweating is a necessary mechanism for maintaining proper heat balance during physical activity. Profuse sweating, however, accomplishes only one thing: a greater-than-normal loss of water from the body. This water loss, if excessive, will make you weigh less temporarily but can cause a dangerous increase in body temperature. A rubber suit, or any uneeded clothing or a hot, humid environment, does not allow the heat produced during exercise to escape from the body. Evaporation of sweat is the major means for heat dissipation at the surface of the skin during vigorous exercise. When you wear a rubber suit, the heat and sweat given off between the suit and the skin are trapped in the suit. The trapped sweat can't evaporate to cool the body.

When the heat produced by the exercising muscles is not eliminated properly, an added burden is imposed on the heat-regulating mechanisms. This leads to a loss of too much body water and, in turn, a decrease in blood volume because of less water in the blood. This causes a severe rise in body temperature and possible circulatory collapse. These events, if severe enough, can produce heat stroke and death.

The key point here is that *dehydration (removal of body water) is useless for weight control and can be dangerous.* You will immediately restore the depleted body water when you eat and drink. Water does not contain calories. Excess body weight (fat) is lost only by burning calories, not by losing water. These weight-reducing practices are not only useless but dangerous, since they can cause the body to become overheated.

A Plan for Losing Weight

If you are overweight and wish to rid your body of excess fat, increasing your physical activity while controlling your food intake is the best method. Striving to be physically fit and maintaining this state of health and well-being over a lifetime increases the possibility of permanent fat loss.

Let's make it clear: weight control is a lifetime concern, not a two-week special diet! It's nonsense to think otherwise. Exercising allows you to burn an extra 300 to 500 calories or more each workout, and that not only helps you lose excess fat but helps you keep it off. Once you have reached your desired weight, being physically active actually allows you to eat better and enjoy some of the foods that inactive people cannot enjoy without facing the consequences of gaining excess weight. It's plain and simple: *Fit people burn more calories because they are more active!*

Setting Goals

It's good to set goals for weight reduction. Before you begin a weight loss program, set up some realistic targets. Determine the number of pounds you need to lose, the number of weeks it will take, and the maximum number of calories you should eat each day.

First you need to determine your ideal or desired weight. In Chapter 5, we presented a simple method for estimating your fat percentage and your ideal weight. Another simple means for estimating your ideal weight is to recall what you weighed in your senior year of high school, assuming you did not have a weight problem at that time. This is as good an estimate as any measurement. Regardless of how you determine your ideal weight, subtract this target value from your present weight. The result is the number of pounds to lose.

Weight reduction should be gradual. Therefore, we suggest dividing the number of excess pounds to lose by one pound, but certainly no more than two pounds, per week. This will give you the number of weeks needed to reach your desired weight. No doubt it will be longer than you'd like, but if you stick to this realistic plan you'll never see these pounds again, providing you remain physically active. A gradual approach is the best approach for keeping excess pounds off permanently.

One key point to remember: expect fluctuations in your weight loss. Some weeks you may be pleasantly surprised by losing more than two pounds; some weeks you may not lose any weight and may even gain a little. However, our experience with people in our program clearly suggests that this system works! No more buying new clothes, then letting them out weeks later, then taking them in again, and so on. Your goal is long-term maintenance of weight control.

You must also determine the maximum daily caloric intake that will enable you to lose your targeted number of pounds. Most people who are moderately active need about 15 calories per pound per day to maintain their weight. If you are moderately active, multiply your present weight by 15 to determine the number of calories needed for your daily activities. A moderately active person weighing 190 pounds will need 2,850 calories a day (15 multiplied by 190). If you sit all day, then a more realistic value is 12 calories per pound of body weight; if you're quite active, a value of 18 calories is reasonable for figuring your daily caloric needs.

There are approximately 3,500 calories in each pound of stored fat. To lose one pound a week, you must reduce your caloric intake by 500 calories a day (3,500 divided by 7). Therefore, for the 190-pound, moderately active person, this means cutting the number of daily calories from 2,850 to 2,350. Given today's choice of readily available foods, this can be difficult. That is why becoming more active in a regular exercise program can be the key to losing weight permanently.

Making It Easier Through Vigorous Exercise

Exercise is often scoffed at as a means of reducing or controlling weight because it requires an energy expenditure of 3,500 calories to lose a pound of fat. Even if you exercised very vigorously for 30 minutes, you would be hard pressed to burn 500 calories. In fact, very few people have this capability, especially when beginning an exercise program. However, if you take a long-range view and exercise at a more reasonable caloric level of 300 calories (a level you can endure) for four days a week, you would be burning an extra 1,200 calories a week. Therefore, if you maintain food intake at a constant level and exercise four days a week, you would lose about one pound every three weeks, or 17 pounds a year.

Now, if you combine vigorous exercise with a cut-back of calories, your probability for shedding excess poundage becomes more favorable and realistic. Again, if you exercise four days a week at 300 calories per session, but also cut your daily food intake by 400 calories (omit two beers and a handful of peanuts), you have a 4,000-calorie deficit per week. Theoretically, this approach would bring about a weight loss of approximately one pound of fat a week. Figure 37 shows some of the possible relationships between daily caloric intake and daily caloric expenditure.

I know what you are going to say, "This one to two pounds a week is too slow!" Believe me, quick and gimmicky diets just don't work in the long run and are unhealthy. You didn't put on this weight over-night, and you are not going to take it off (permanently) overnight. Naturally you are eager to lose weight, but the process has to be slow if the weight is to stay off. Body weight lost gradually (no more than two pounds a week) and systematically has a greater tendency to stay off.

The minimal threshold for weight reduction and fat loss through vigorous endurance-type exercise alone involves working out for four days a week for 30 minutes. Since energy expenditure can cause a re-duction in fat, increasing the frequency, intensity, and duration of your workout can yield greater reduction.

Let's look ahead for a moment. Most likely if you have a weight problem, you have been inactive. I would first recommend that you follow the walking charts suggested in Chapter 8. Not only will you become more fit as you proceed through the charts, but you will begin burning a higher rate of calories. You will probably start walking for 20 minutes at first. Depending on your walking pace and your weight, this will only result in burning 100 to 150 calories. Once you can walk longer (45 minutes to an hour) you will be burning closer to 300 calories or more. Eventually you will be able to walk faster, burn a higher rate of calories (you're becoming more fit), and even be able to increase the intensity of your workouts by incorporating some short running bouts with your walking (see Chapter 9). To repeat, the more fit you become, the more calories you can burn over a similar time period. As you progress, you may be able to sustain a running workout for 30 minutes, with the potential of burning 350 to 400 calories or more. If you become fit enough to run for an hour you can double this energy expenditure to between 700 and 800 calories. This is why being fit greatly helps you control your body weight.

When we walk, run, swim, or cycle, some remarkable things hap-pen. We feel better, look better, have more energy, and can control our weight better. Proper exercise on a regular basis is the best way to achieve lifelong weight control.

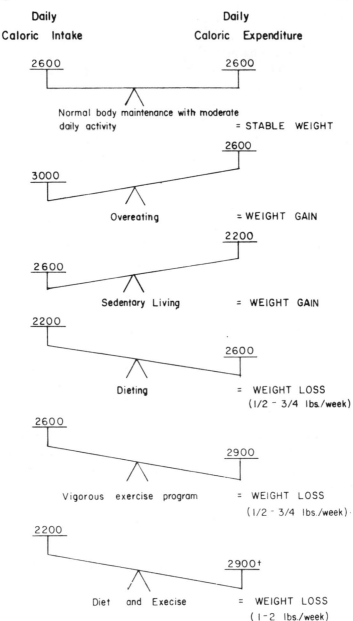

Daily
Caloric Intake

Daily
Caloric Expenditure

2600   2600

Normal body maintenance with moderate
daily activity   = STABLE WEIGHT

3000   2600

Overeating   = WEIGHT GAIN

2600   2200

Sedentary Living   = WEIGHT GAIN

2200   2600

Dieting   = WEIGHT LOSS
                              (1/2 - 3/4 lbs./week)

2600   2900

Vigorous exercise program   = WEIGHT LOSS
                              (1/2 - 3/4 lbs./week)

2200   2900†

Diet and Execise   = WEIGHT LOSS
                              (1-2 lbs./week)

Figure 37.

What About a Special Diet?

For some, in order to be successful in losing weight, it helps to follow a planned diet. However, stay away from severe caloric restrictions and suspect any diet that eliminates any nutrients. Many people have joined the Weight Watchers International and benefited from its weekly motivational sessions and diet plans. Such a program may help you at first, but eventually you have to learn to manage your personal nutrition yourself. I suggest that you learn more about the nutrient content of foods and study nutrition just as you have been studying exercise in this book. Learn the caloric values of food and watch for hidden and empty calories. Although I don't like the word "diet," a planned program of eating may be necessary to start you on a weight control program. But as with the exercise charts, eventually you won't need to follow a planned diet every day. Your exercise and eating habits will become an integral part of your everyday living.

Changing Your Lifestyle

By now I hope you realize that losing weight involves changing your lifestyle. Since being overweight is the result of improper eating and activity habits practiced for years, both of these behaviors must be changed if weight is to be lost. This adjustment in behavior cannot be accomplished overnight. Drastic changes or crash diet programs usually fail.

Often the people who come to our physical fitness program at Ball State have been shopping for an easy and magical way to lose weight. After much frustration with special diets and exercise gimmicks (vacupants, the bull worker, and so on) they decide to try vigorous exercise as a last resort. It's necessary to recognize and accept the fact that there is no magical formula or easy way to lose weight. It is hard work to change eating patterns and include exercise in your life.

The first and most important change is to become more active. There are thousands of formerly fat people walking through our parks, running through our streets, swimming in our lakes and pools, and skiing across our mountains. Often, just an increase in their activity habits made the difference. For some, an adjustment in their eating habits may also have been necessary.

So, first begin an exercise program. Once you become accustomed to exercising, you can begin to make dietary changes. It's tough to become a different person overnight. Go one step at a time. It takes patience and persistence.

There has been much interest in the use of behavior modification procedures in recent years for treating weight problems. Professors Richard Carr and Judy Roepke of the Family Nutrition Education Center at Ball State and I work closely with people in our program who have serious weight problems and want special help. Two hours a week group meetings are held along with attendance at the four morning exercise sessions. The group meeting deals with nutrition, diet, and behavior modification. Each participant's physical condition is assessed and an individualized exercise program and diet is designed. Here are some of the behavior modification guidelines that we use in our weight management program to help people change inappropriate eating habits.

1. Begin by observing your eating habits for a week or two. Write down what you eat, when, where, and how much, then ask yourself why you ate it. Reading your diary at the end of the week may surprise you. Understanding your eating habits is half the battle.

2. Separate your eating from other behaviors. Don't eat on the run, in front of the TV, or in the bedroom; when you eat — *eat* — don't do anything else while you enjoy your food. Stick to one place — the kitchen or dining room. You will be amazed at the number of calories this change will save you.

3. Put a serving of food on your plate, then put away leftovers before you sit down. This makes it tougher to get extra helpings.

4. Buy groceries on a full stomach. This prevents impulse buying. Don't buy the junk foods you crave. This is tough, but if you don't buy them, you can't eat them.

5. Eat slowly. Chewing at a rate of one crunch per minute is carrying it a little far, but slowing down gives your digestive system time to let your brain know that food's being received. It takes about 20 minutes for food to get into your blood stream and turn off your hunger pangs.

6. Make it a family affair, if you can. The dietary habits of the whole family will benefit. Most likely, other members of your family have developed some poor nutritional habits.

These suggestions are based on the assumption that improper eating habits can be changed. Excessive eating is a strongly conditioned response to numerous everyday surroundings and emotional stimuli. The cues for food are all quite familiar: sitting in front of the television, being with friends and family, feeling angry, happy, lonely, or bored. All of us will occasionally wolf down a carton of ice cream or a bag of cookies when the mood strikes us. Breaking such lifelong habits is not easy.

Summary

We live in a society that has become increasingly inactive with the advancement of technology. Today, sedentary living is being encouraged by the continued development of automated work-savers and the promotion of passive amusements and recreation. Considering our plentiful but often poor diet, as well as the daily tensions characteristic of modern times, we see dismal prospects for maintaining an optimal level of health and appearance. The human body was made to be active, and it thrives on movement and vigorous activity. The ability to sit all day without getting fat was not bred into our bodies.

Obesity and inactivity have been correlated with coronary heart disease, high blood pressure, diabetes, and other degenerative disorders. But obesity and fatness are practically unknown among vigorous, active people. This is because *exercise is the key factor in controlling weight*. A sound, nutritious diet combined with regular vigorous exercise is the best strategy for a lifetime of successful weight control. The goal is not merely to lose fat, but to keep it off, or better still, never put it on. Now is the time to establish sound nutritional and exercise habits.

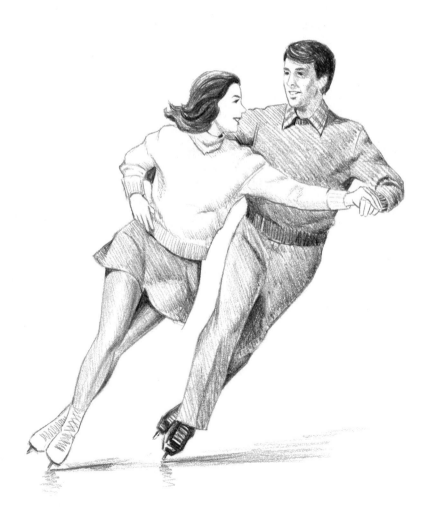

chapter fifteen

Getting the Most Out of Sports

Sports are played for fun, not for fitness. It is traditionally assumed that playing sports is a way of improving your level of physical fitness and, consequently, your general health. Some people think you can even "play" yourself into good physical condition. In most cases, this is not true. The top athletes train vigorously in order to play their specialty. It's common for teams as well as individuals to devote a significant block of time for warming up in order to stretch key muscles to avoid injuries during practice or competitions. It is also quite common for athletes to engage in individual running and weight lifting programs to better prepare themselves for the actual playing of their sport. The same holds true for the average sports participant: *You need to get in shape to play sports, rather than play sports to get in shape.* Being physically fit to play sports means getting more enjoyment out of your play.

Most sports — team or individual — do not provide sufficient rhythmic endurance-type movement to develop and maintain cardiorespiratory fitness. But, regular participation in some sports, complements your fitness conditioning program. Sports that require speed and skills provide an important dimension to all-round fitness development. The movements required in the racket sports (badminton, tennis, racquetball, squash) are lacking in running, cycling, and other cardiorespiratory developers.

As a general rule, the longer and more continuous a sport is played, the greater the cardiorespiratory benefits. In contrast, sports involving short bursts of movement followed by varying periods of rest do little for developing cardiorespiratory fitness.

The above can be illustrated when we study maximal oxygen uptakes (aerobic capacities) of elite athletes. Long-distance runners, cross-country skiers, swimmers, and other such endurance athletes have significantly higher average values (70 to 80 ml/kg·min) than football players, baseball players, gymnasts, and other top athletes from sports characterized by short bouts of explosive play. In fact, the latter group of athletes show average maximal oxygen uptake values ranging from 48 ml/kg·min to values in the low 50s — only slightly above average for non-athletes. Players from sports that represent a combination of fitness requirements (short bursts and continuous and rhythmical exertions) will range in the high 50s to low 60s. These athletes represent such sports as soccer, field hockey, basketball, and tennis. These measurements tend to indicate what sports can provide cardiorespiratory benefits.

An interesting story comes to mind about an avid tennis player in our community who we tested in 1968. His maximal oxygen uptake was 38 ml/kg·min — an average value for his age. At that time I encouraged him to begin running to improve his physical fitness, in order to establish a better physiological base for his tennis game. He was hesitant at that time, but within the last five years he has progressed to the point were he now runs four to six miles each workout. Just last year we tested him and his maximal oxygen uptake value was at 55 ml/kg·min, an impressive level. When discussing this with Dick, he was quick to point out the importance of his regular running to his tennis game. "Not only am I in better shape, but my tennis is much more fun."

Important Considerations

Throughout this book I have emphasized the importance of following a regular schedule (four times a week, at least) of vigorous health-promoting exercise. The availability of facilities is just one of the problems of establishing a regular routine for playing sports for fitness. A simple racquetball match becomes complicated by such details as scheduling a court, finding an opponent, and setting the time that fits your schedule. If it is a seasonal outdoor sport, bad weather can spoil the best made plans. Most sports are not suitable for daily or four-time-a-week programs. Still, they can provide a welcome break from your regular workouts, and an added bonus to your fitness program.

Keep in mind that the benefits from sports participation vary from person to person. Any attempt to rate and compare the sports as to their relative contribution to developing physical fitness can be questioned. To date, there is only limited research to support such judgments. The intensity of a player's activity and the energy required varies according to age, skills, and fitness level, and in team sports, the skill of other players. Therefore the energy cost values for sports are not as exact as we would like. Nevertheless, we have developed the following table, which includes energy cost ratings that are based on our own as well as others' research. For each sport listed, we give a MET range and a range of estimated caloric values. The exact amount of energy (calories) depends on how much you weigh as well as how vigorously you play. Qualifying words (i.e., excellent, good, fair, poor) as to the overall potential of each sport as a fitness developer are provided to help you to make comparisons. What is most important is how demanding these sports are on the body. In other words, what are the specific physiological requirements of each?

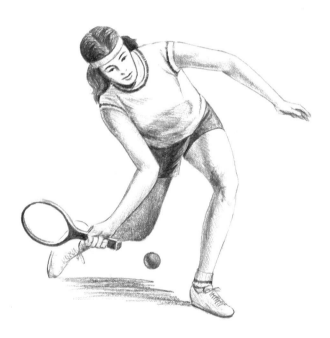

For an example, let's look at racquetball. It's a sport that most people can play with reasonable success after brief instruction and practice. How does it rate as a fitness activity? Racquetball is vigorous; it uses big muscles; it requires high levels of energy and, it is generally played for at least an hour. It is not played continuously but intermittently with brief stops in between serves. Successful play is highly

FITNESS POTENTIAL FOR POPULAR SPORTS

SPORT	CARDIORESPIRATORY ENDURANCE	MUSCULAR STRENGTH & ENDURANCE UPPER BODY	MUSCULAR STRENGTH & ENDURANCE LOWER BODY	FLEXIBILITY	MET RANGE	CAL/MIN	CALORIC RANGE CAL/HOUR
Back packing[1]	Good to Fair	Fair	Good	Fair	4-8	5-10	300-600
Badminton	Good to Fair	Fair	Fair	Fair	4-8	5-10	300-600
Baseball/Softball	Fair to Poor	Fair	Fair	Fair	3-6	4-7.5	240-450
Basketball	Good	Fair	Good	Fair	8-10	10-12.5	600-750
Bowling	Poor	Fair	Poor	Poor	2-3	2.5-4	150-240
Canoeing	Good to Fair	Good	Poor	Poor	3-8	4-10	240-600
Football (touch)	Fair to Poor	Fair	Fair	Fair	4-8	5-10	300-600
Golf	Poor	Fair	Good	Fair	3-4	4-5	240-300
Handball	Good	Good	Good	Fair	6-12	10-12.5	600-750
Karate	Fair	Good	Good	Excellent	6-8	7.5-10	450-600
Racquetball	Good	Good	Good	Fair	6-10	7.5-12.5	450-750
Scuba diving	Poor	Fair	Fair	Fair	4-6	5-7.5	300-450
Skating (ice)	Good to Fair	Poor	Good-Fair	Fair	4-8	5-10	300-600

FITNESS POTENTIAL FOR POPULAR SPORTS (continued)

SPORT	CARDIORESPIRATORY ENDURANCE	MUSCULAR STRENGTH & ENDURANCE		FLEXIBILITY	MET RANGE	CAL/MIN	CALORIC RANGE CAL/HOUR
		UPPER BODY	LOWER BODY				
Skating (roller)	Good to Fair	Poor	Good–Fair	Fair	4–8	5–10	300–600
Skiing (alpine)	Fair	Good	Good	Good	5–9	6–10	360–600
Skiing (nordic)	Excellent–Good	Good	Excellent	Good	6–12	7.5–15	450–900
Soccer	Good–Excellent	Fair	Good–Excellent	Good	6–12	7.5–15	450–900
Surfing[2]	Good[2]	Good	Good	Good	4–10	5–12.5	300–750
Tennis	Good–Fair	Good–Fair	Good	Fair	4–8	5–10	300–600
Volleyball	Good–Fair	Fair	Good–Fair	Fair	4–8	5–10	300–600
Waterskiing	Poor	Good	Good	Fair	4–6	5–7.5	300–450

[1] Benefits depend on walking terrain and weight of pack.
[2] Paddling the board out beyond the breaking waves can be demanding.

dependent on the functional ability of your heart and aerobic systems. It does require strength, particularly the ability to sustain strength — muscular endurance. Range of motion-flexibility is quite specific as similar muscular movements are repeated constantly. Therefore, as the chart indicates, racquetball rates good on cardiorespiratory endurance, muscular strength and endurance (upper and lower body), and fair to good on flexibility. Keep in mind these ratings are based on the average participant rather than the expert player. Generally the energy required to play racquetball properly can range from as low as 8 METs to as high as 12 METs. The reason for this wide range is the variance of both the skill and the fitness capabilities of the participant. To put it another way, 8 METs, when expressed as maximal fitness, is considered low for active people. One needs a 10- or 11-MET max to be able to perform an activity at an 8 MET level. On the other end of the scale, if you are capable of playing racquetball at a 12-MET level, this requires a high fitness capacity of 15 to 16 METs. This example further clarifies the point that *you need to get in shape so you can play to the fullest your favorite sport.* The better your condition, the better your chance of getting a good workout when playing sports. If you presently possess a low level of fitness, investing significant amounts of time playing racquetball or any other sport for developing fitness is questionable. First, involve your total body in sustained vigorous exercise so you can develop your heart, lungs, and muscles so you fully enjoy the maximal benefits from sports participation.

Let's look at golf. I personally spent over two years studying the fitness and energy responses of people who play golf. In 1968, when I presented my data at a National meeting in Chicago, one of my conclusions based on the data presented was that "golf is not a suitable activity for developing fitness." Comparisons were made on over 30 fitness measurements on 20 middle-age male golfers and, with similar groups of controls such as non-golfers and runners (8 to 12 miles a week). The controls and golfers were very inactive prior to the golf season when they were first tested. When retested in early September each golfer felt he was in better shape, but only one of the measurements showed improvement when compared to the control group. The golfer's leg strength increased significantly. The cardiorespiratory measures did not improve. When compared to the running program group, vast differences in cardiorespiratory fitness resulted. Also, extensive energy-cost studies were completed on four of these men. The results, which have been published, showed the average energy requirement for golf to be about three times that of sitting in a chair (3 METs). I personally enjoy playing golf, so my intentions were not to discredit the sport, but as this study indicated, the exercise requirements of golf (both energy cost and heart rate stimulation) were not adequate for fitness gains.

Summary

I encourage you to complement your personal fitness training by getting involved in the playing of sports. But first get in shape. Many of the people in our program at Ball State have discovered new sports horizons in their lives. To their benefit and pleasure they have found that being fit opened up possibilities in sports they never thought possible. Participating in sports is another way to enjoy the pleasures of being physically fit.

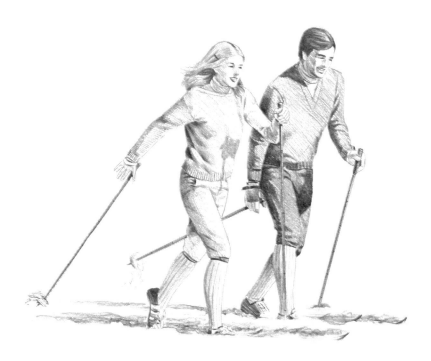

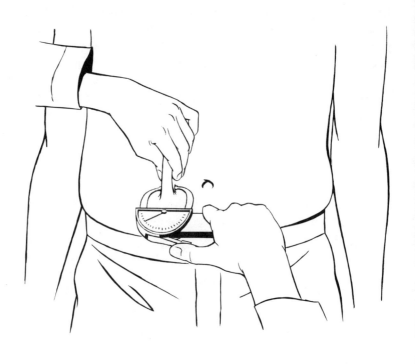

Measuring Skinfolds to Estimate Body Fat

Measuring skinfold thickness is considered to be an acceptable method for estimating the amount of fat on one's body. Research studies indicate that this technique correlates well with the underwater weighing technique — an elaborate laboratory method for determining body fat. In addition, measuring skinfolds is more practical for testing large groups. The calipers are inexpensive, measurements can easily be made, and estimates quickly calculated. Most testing centers have skinfold calipers and utilize an acceptable formula for determining your fat percentage. Recently, companies are providing inexpensive calipers for purchase (see list of sources).

Dr. A.W. Sloan and his fellow researchers have developed formulas using skinfold measurements as predictors. For men, the fat thickness at the subscapula and thigh sites have proven to be a good gauge of overall body fatness. For women, the triceps and suprailiac sites tend to be good predictors.

Below are the proper methods of measuring skinfolds with calipers, along with the nomograms for estimating your fat.

Procedure: (See Figure 38.)
1. First, you need someone to measure you.
2. Skinfolds are measured on the right side of the body using the skinfold caliper.
3. Grasp the skinfold between thumb and forefinger. The skinfold should include two thicknesses of skin and subcutaneous fat, but not muscle.
4. Apply the calipers just below the fingers holding the skinfold, at a depth equal to the thickness of the fold.

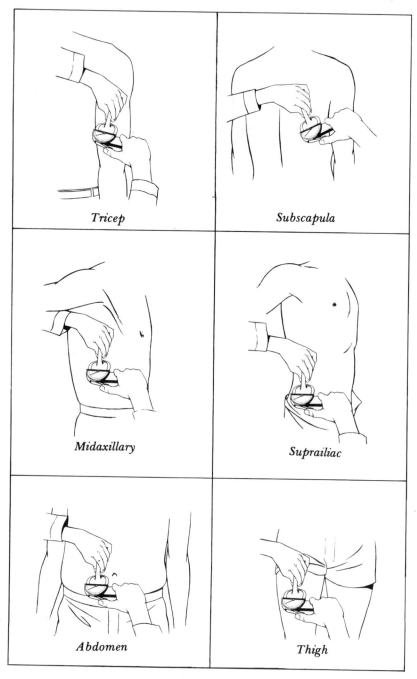

Figure 38.

5. Each fold is taken in the vertical plane while the subject is standing, except for the subscapular and suprailiac, which are picked up on a slight slant running laterally with the natural fold of the skin.

6. The technique of measurement is repeated completely for each site before going on to the next site. This includes regrasping the skinfold. Whenever there is a difference greater than 0.5 millimeter, a third measurement is necessary. The mean of the two closest readings represents the value for the site being measured.

7. The anatomical landmarks for six skinfold sites are as follows:
   1. Triceps
        The back of the upper arm midway between the shoulder and elbow joints.
   2. Subscapula
        The bottom point of the shoulder blade (scapula).
   3. Midaxillary
        The middle of the side on the level with the lower end of the sternum.
   4. Suprailiac
        Just above the top of the hip bone (crest of the ilium) at the middle of the side of the body.
   5. Abdomen
        Approximately two centimeters (one inch) to the side of your navel.
   6. Thigh
        The middle front side of the thigh midway between the hip and knee joints.

Nomograms for Predicting Body Fat

Your percentage of body fats can be quickly assessed from the following graphs. A straight line joining your skinfold value will intersect your value for percentage of fat.

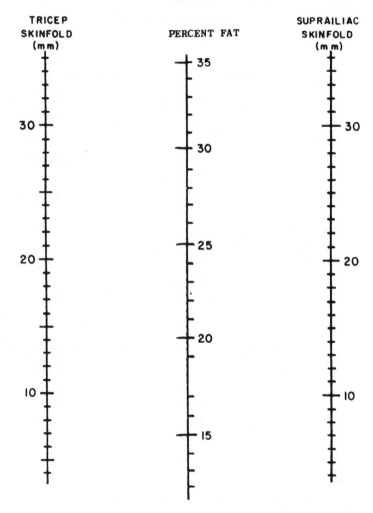

PERCENT. BODY FAT

WOMEN

TRICEP
SKINFOLD
(mm)

PERCENT FAT

SUPRAILIAC
SKINFOLD
(mm)

NOMOGRAM FOR CONVERSION OF SKINFOLDS
TO PERCENT BODY FAT

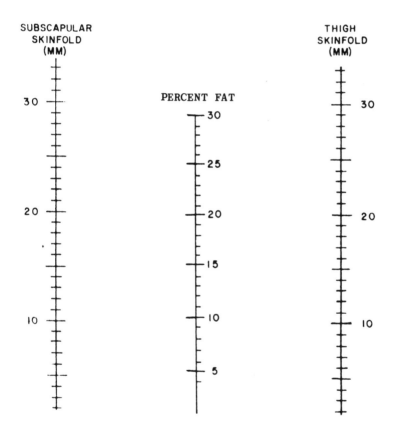

PERCENT BODY FAT

MEN

SUBSCAPULAR
SKINFOLD
(MM)

PERCENT FAT

THIGH
SKINFOLD
(MM)

**NOMOGRAM FOR CONVERSION OF SKINFOLDS
TO PERCENT BODY FAT**

Body Fat Norms

The chart below is also presented in Chapter 5. This body fat classification chart provides you with ratings for both men and women. Remember, a normal rating refers to the average for the group that was measured. This does not necessarily mean that this is the most desired rating. As referred to earlier, desired percentages of body fat for men and women range from 10 to 12% and 18 to 20%, respectively.

BODY FAT NORMS

CLASSIFICATION	WOMAN%	MEN%
Very low fat: skinny	14.0-16.9	7.0-9.9
Low fat: trim	17.0-19.9	10.0-12.9
Average fat: normal	20.0-23.9	13.0-16.9
Above normal fat: plump	24.0-26.9	17.0-19.9
Very high fat: fat	27.0-29.9	20.0-24.9
Obese: over fat	30.0 and higher	25.0 and higher

Sum of Six Skinfolds

Another interesting way to analyze your body fat is to look at the sum of your skinfolds. A measurement of 25 millimeters (mm) is approximately one inch. As a rule, an inch or more of fat at one of the sites indicates too much fat. A better value would be in the range of ½ inch, or 12 to 13 mm. When the six values are added, a total score of 75 mm and below indicates trimness; 75 to 100 mm would be a reasonably good score; a range of 100 to 140 mm indicates some flabbiness; and over 140 mm generally indicates too much fat. Observing each value individually can provide easy identification of areas of too much fat.

Determining a Desirable Weight

The following procedures represent a simple way of determining an effective weight for you based on your present *fat free weight*. For example, let's say a man weighs 200 pounds and his skinfold measures indicate a body fat of 20%. This calculates to 40 pounds of fat weight (20% of 200), or a fat-free weight (lean body weight) of 160 pounds (200 − 40). The latter figure is not his ideal weight, however, because no body can or should be completely free of fat. Referring to the body fat norms, we can take 12% as a desirable body fat level for men. With this figure we can estimate the weight that corresponds to this selected percentage of body fat. In this case, just divide the fat-free weight by 0.88 (100% − 12.0% or 1.00 − 0.12). The result, in this example, computes to just under 182 pounds (82 kg).

This procedure implies that a weight of 182 pounds represents a reasonable goal for the man in our example. For those who have a very high fat percentage, 17.5% or 15% might be a more appropriate first goal. For women we suggest a 18% value as a desirable goal when using the Sloan formula. In this case, the fat-free weight should be divided by 0.82. Below is an example of the computation steps for a 145-pound woman who predicted 28.3% body fat.

Example for Calculating "Desired" Weight.
Computation:

1. Fat Weight = Weight × $\dfrac{\% \text{ Fat}}{100}$

   = $\underline{145}$ × $\underline{.283}$ = $\underline{41.0}$ lbs.

2. Fat-free Weight = Weight − Fat Weight

   = $\underline{145}$ − 41 = $\underline{104}$ lbs. (46.8 kg.)

3. Desired Weight at 18% Fat = Fat-free Weight ÷ 0.82

   = $\underline{104}$ ÷ 0.82

   Desired Weight = $\underline{126.8}$ lbs.

Sources for Skinfold Calipers

The three skinfold calipers below represent attempts to produce inexpensive devices for measuring fat. These appear to be quite satisfactory in helping you evaluate your body fat.

Fat-O-Meter—Health Education Services Corp., 7N015 York Rd., Bensenville, IL 60106 (312) 766-6655. $9.95*

Slim Guide—Creative Health Products, 9135 General Ct., Plymouth, MI 48170. (313) 453-5309. $19.95*

Fat Control—Fat Control, Inc., P.O. Box 10117, Towson, MD 21204. $7.95*

The calipers below are made for testing centers and research labs. Due to cost, they are not practical for home use.

Lange—Cambridge Scientific Industries, Inc., Cambridge, MD. $172.25*

Harpendon—Quinton Instrument Co., 2121 Terry Ave., Seattle, WA 98121. (206) 223-7373. $197.50*

*Prices subject to change.

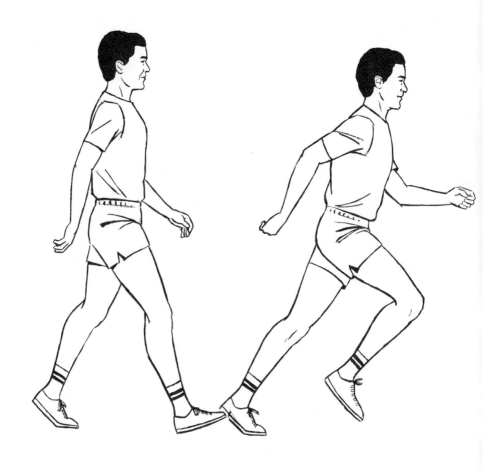

Appendix B

Selecting Proper Footwear for Walking and Running

For fitness walking and running, it is important to buy a pair of good sturdy shoes that fit properly. Most running shoes are suitable for walking. There are many fine shoes available today with good multilayered spongelike soles and a strong heel counter. However, be cautious for the so-called "running shoes" that sell at bargain prices. Most of these are of poor quality and everything from blisters to shin splints may be part of the bargain. Your best bet is to buy shoes from a reputable sporting goods store. The purchase of quality shoes can be a wise investment. The properly made training shoe must function to support the foot and be able to absorb shock so as to protect you from injury. Above all, the shoes must fit you properly and be comfortable. Before you buy, check to see if it is built like the one in the illustration below. Take a moment to become familiar with the parts of the shoe.

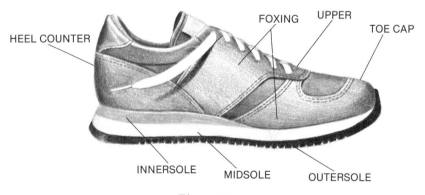

Figure 39.

1. Outersole—the bottom of the shoe that makes contact with the ground—a durable, flexible, lightweight material. Common types are waffle, ripple, and cross ridges.

2. Midsole (wedge)—portion of the shoe between the outer sole and insole. This elevates the heel, reduces shock to the heel, and helps keep the weight forward.

3. Innersole—the inner soft portion of the shoe that the foot rests on.

4. Heel counter—inflexible molded material that cradles the heel to prevent rotation and lateral slippage of the heel.

5. Toe cap—designed to give toes room to move and help prevent blisters.

6. Upper—the material covering the upper part of the shoe. Nylon is preferred.

7. Foxing—additional material added to strategic places to give added support and looks to the shoe.

Proper Fitting

1. Always take the measurements for size while standing, and if possible, near the end of the day when your feet are slightly larger.

2. Fit the shoe from heel to toe length first. If you have a second toe longer than your big toe (called Morton's toe) measure from the end of that toe. The width is measured at the ball of the foot at the widest part. The heel should fit snugly.

3. The sole (outer sole and midsole) should allow flexibility while providing good cushioning. The forefoot area must be flexible, especially under the ball of the foot where the shoe will bend. This flexibility is essential for ease in pushing off. To test for flexibility, hold the shoe in your hands and bend the toe box and forefoot area of shoe back toward the heel. It should bend easily but not all the way back to touch the shoe laces. Extreme stiffness should be avoided.

4. A very important characteristic of a good shoe is the heel counter. It should be constructed of a rigid material.

5. Be sure you allow enough room for your toes. A roomy toe box keeps the upper material from rubbing the tops of the toes. Allow for *at least* 1/4-inch extra toe length.

6. Be sure to try on and test various brands and models. Walk around in them.

7. Buy shoes that have a good reputation. Most stores that specialize in running shoes have trained sales persons to assist you. Most important, buy shoes that feel the best to you after they have met the specifications mentioned above.

About the Authors

Bud Getchell was born in Malden, Massachusetts and graduated from Springfield College in 1955. As a college athlete he was selected by the American Association of College Baseball Coaches as an All-American second baseman in 1955. He has coached both baseball and basketball on the collegiate level. He earned his Ph.D. at the University of Illinois under the tutelage of Dr. Thomas K. Cureton, a pioneer in the area of physical fitness.

At Ball State University, Dr. Getchell initiated the Human Performance Laboratory and the Adult Physical Fitness Program in 1965. This program has grown to be recognized nationwide as one of the most successful ongoing physical fitness programs and the Human Performance Laboratory, under the direction of Dr. David Costill, is now recognized as one of the leading exercise laboratories in the world.

Bud Getchell is a Fellow and serves on the Board of Trustees of the American College of Sports Medicine (ACSM). He is a certified Rehabilitative and Preventive Exercise Program Director and a past president of the Midwest Chapter of ACSM. He lectures extensively at research and medical meetings, wellness conferences, physical fitness workshops, and was speaker at the Second White House Conference on Physical Fitness. His writings include contributions to a variety of research, medical, and sports publications. Hundreds of universities use his text *Physical Fitness: A Way of Life.*

Wayne Anderson was born in Petersburg, Virginia and received his Master of Arts in Education in 1968 from Princeton Seminary. He has over fourteen years experience in educational publishing as marketer and editor for John Wiley & Sons.

About the Artist

Keith Freeman, a successful commercial artist for most of his career, has in recent years devoted his talents almost exclusively to wildlife illustration. His sharp eye for detail and flawless techniques can be measured not only in this work, but in the many private and public collections which now display his work.

Mr. Freeman attended the Corcoran Art School, Washington, D.C., the Meintzinger Art School, Detroit, and the Art Center School, Los Angeles, where he began his professional career. His works have been published in numerous popular calendar series and the WORLD BOOK ENCYCLOPEDIA.

Index